Mikhail Tombak, Ph.D.

Can We Live 150 Years?

Your Body Maintenance Handbook

Second English Edition

Healthy Life Press Inc.

Translated by Jan Madejski

Disclaimer
Any suggestions for techniques, treatments, or lifestyle change described in this book should be used at the reader's discretion under the guidance of a licensed therapist or health-care practitioner. The author, editors, translator and publisher disclaim any and all liability arising directly or indirectly from the use of any information contained in this book.

Translated by: Jan Madejski
Cover and Illustrations: Luke Zukowski
Typesetting: Robert Borowski, Stanislaw Wnuk

Published by
Healthy Life Press Inc.
145 Tyee Drive, PMB 355
Point Roberts, WA 98281-9602
USA
http://www.starthealthylife.com
info@starthealthylife.com
Tel. (888) 575-3173
Tel. (604) 468-1213

Second English Edition
First edition 2003
Second edition 2005

ISBN: 978-0-9727328-4-0
LCCN: 2005931849

Printed in Canada

Contents

Part Two

Healthy Spine – The Foundation of a Healthy Body

Part Three

Obesity – Your Worst Enemy

Part Four

"Natural Doctors" Who Are Always with You

Part Five

Some Food for Thought

Part Six

Complete Body Cleansing

Part Seven

Health without Medications
Folk Medicine Formulas

From the publisher

Much has been written lately about ways to attain long and healthy life. Numerous miracle diets are presented, formulas are praised for their extraordinary qualities, weight-reduction and aging-reversal methods are advertised. People are led to believe that good health may be the result of taking a miraculous pill. In reality, return to full health requires many years of effort, just as our diseases are caused by many years of neglect. Full health does not depend on miraculous medication and formulas that cause weight loss or aging reversal, but on the lifestyle that is in harmony with nature. This philosophy permeates the contents of this book. The author of this book, Mikhail Tombak, created a holistic system of maintaining good health.

The book does not contain miraculous diets; it contains simple principles of maintaining and protecting our health. There is no requirement of strict calorie counting but there are simple, obvious, and natural nutritional principles.

The author emphasizes a close connection between our health and the way we eat, breathe, and take care of all our physical and psychological needs. The question is not limited only to nutrition as is the case with many dieting programs.

As we worked on preparing this book, we were pleasantly surprised by the author's humble personality. He does not like to talk about his successes or the ways he has achieved them. According to him, the merit of his health maintenance system finds its best expression in the testimony of people who applied it in their life. This quality shows in the following fragment of his interview with the editorial team prior to publishing:

> *When people ask me about success stories, I have one answer – It would be easy to boast, but the real criterion is the way my work is judged by others. They give testimony based on their experience and changes in the condition of their health.*
>
> *If the system I write about were not effective, people would not be buying my books. They have been among top bestselling books for the last five years.*
>
> *More and more readers understand my philosophy of health maintenance. They believed in my methods and became finally convinced when they observed these simple methods work very effectively in changing the health con-*

dition of their own bodies. They tell success stories to their relatives and friends, increasing the circle of people who favor natural healing methods.

My task is simply to help people realize that nobody is able to outsmart nature.

The most interesting conclusion from the reading of this book is contained in a known idea: Our health is in our own hands. Moreover, the therapies are non-invasive and can be done at home without any help, using natural and widely available ingredients without the typical arsenal of pharmaceuticals.

The book also contains some unusual, even shocking, but extremely effective methods of body cleansing. They are based on millennia-old traditions of Eastern and Western natural medicine, but they are ignored by modern mainstream medicine.

We invite you to enjoy this book.

To my readers:

The author realizes that the contents of this book, concerning practically all aspects of the human body, cannot be free of controversy. It is understandable that experts can point out flaws of arguments and insufficient accuracy of details – I wrote this book with the wide general public in mind.

I would like to turn your attention to the fact that we know very little about our body and its close relationship with the natural environment. Our future life often depends on the method of treatment we choose in a case of a health crisis. In cases when mainstream medicine cannot offer any help, we should remember that there are natural therapies that can prove themselves very effective.

I am deeply convinced that we should be our own advisor and doctor in many situations. We need to attain enough knowledge about the way our body functions to be capable of eliminating the causes of our illness and suffering.

If, as a result of my advice, some people start feeling better, some get cured, and some realize the necessity of health maintenance, the objective of this book will be fulfilled.

I have tried many methods and remedies in my practice and selected those, which are indeed valuable and effective. They are presented here for you to explore. Please use them wisely.

I wish you good health,

Mikhail Tombak

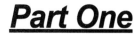
Part One

FIVE FACTORS CAUSING DAMAGE TO OUR HEALTH

Can we live to be 150 years old?

According to the principles of ancient Chinese medicine (confirmed by recent scientific research), our body is a big energy system with cells and organs closely interconnected by energy flowing along twelve energy conduits. Each of us has a few kinds of energy, undergoing constant change and transformation from one type into another.

Energy forms a biological layer around our body – an "aura" – which determines our physical and psychological condition.

A complete cycle of energy exchange in our body lasts seven years. There are 22 such cycles in our life, which means that from the point of view of accumulated energy, we should live about 150 years.

Skeptics may say that 150 years is an exaggeration. Nevertheless, we have an opportunity to live a long life and, what is even more important, to stay healthy.

Our body ages and becomes ill when the balance between its healthy cells and its ill cells is shifted in favor of the latter. To stop aging means to change this unfavorable balance. Theoretically, if we create proper circumstances for that process, our cells are able to completely repair themselves within a seven-year period.

Science proves that we inherit 15% of our health from our parents, another 15% can be influenced by doctors, but the remaining 70% depends only on our lifestyle.

This is why I suggest analyzing together a series of lifestyle errors that lead us to illness and premature aging.

I have read numerous books about the essence of health and illness and helped many people to return to their physical fitness and overall wellbeing.

Based on experience, I have determined that there are five main factors causing damage to our health:

    I. **NEGLECTED SPINE**
   II. **INCORRECT BREATHING**
  III. **INCORRECT DIET**
  IV. **LACK OF INTERNAL BODY HYGIENE**
   V. **INABILITY TO LIVE A BLISSFUL LIFE**

NEGLECTED SPINE

Stand in front of a mirror and take a close look at yourself. What is your spine like? Is your back becoming hunched? Does your abdomen push forward? Do you suffer from back pains?

Unfortunately, most people have these symptoms because they have weak back muscles. They used to hold our spine without much strain. Our muscles become weak as we age, mainly as a result of physical inactivity, incorrect diet, obesity, sleeping on soft mattresses, etc.

An ill spine means an ill body

I once had a 35-year-old female patient suffering from persistent headaches. She also had the feeling of heaviness in the heart area, and any kind of physical effort made her tired. When I examined her, I noticed dislocated cervical vertebrae.

Another female patient suffered from insomnia and stomach pain. The cause of her condition was also a slight dislocation of the cervical and thoracic vertebrae. In both cases, an adjustment of the vertebrae removed the symptoms. I would like to add that both ladies had earlier done X-ray pictures, and they did not show any changes in their spines.

Why am I bringing up these examples? Sometimes the best methods of examination are unable to detect minute dislocations of vertebrae, causing symptoms that have apparently nothing to do with our spine.

Our spine is the column that supports everything our body consists of. Various movements can often cause minute dislocations of vertebrae; the muscles around a dislocated vertebra stiffen up and prevent it from moving back to its proper position. This results in progressive nerve and muscle inflammation, causing pain and limiting our range of motion.

A dislocated vertebra creates pressure on nerves and blood vessels that are connected with specific muscles and organs. **If a nerve remains under pressure for a long time, the organ depending on that nerve develops pathologies that are hard to cure.**

See Table 1 for examples.

Table 1

Misalignment of vertebrae	Problems caused
Cervical	Allergies, loss of hearing, sight problems, eczema, throat problems, thyroid gland disorders
Thoracic	Asthma, pain in the lower arms, back pains, gall bladder disorders, liver problems, stomach and duodenum ulcers, kidney diseases, skin disorders (acne, rashes, eczema, boils)
Lumbar	Hemorrhoids, bladder disorders, irregular menstrual cycle, menstrual pains, impotence, knee pain, lumbago, lumbar pain, poor blood circulation in the legs, ankle swelling, cold feet, weak legs, muscular spasms in the legs

This is still an incomplete list of disorders that could be caused by neglecting our spine.

According to statistics, one out of ten children in the world wears glasses, suffers from allergies, frequent headaches, abdominal pain, chronic colds, attention deficit, etc. The cause of these problems, and many others among the younger generation, is a degenerated spine. We neglect it from early childhood without realizing that it will cause most of our health problems when we become adults.

This is why, in order to return to good health, we should first start paying attention to our spine.

You can find some advice on how to do it in the chapter "Healthy Spine."

INCORRECT BREATHING

When we come into this world, the first thing we do is to take a deep breath. The last thing we do leaving the world is to stop breath-

17

ing. **Our life is what occurs between our birth and death, and it depends completely on our breathing. Breathing is the invisible "food," without which we cannot live for even five minutes.** Some German studies suggest that as many as nine out of ten people breathe incorrectly. Why is this happening?

Try watching little children breathe. Their abdomens expand and contract as they breathe in and out, utilizing especially a major muscle called the **diaphragm.** With this kind of breathing, the lungs have a lot of room to take air into their middle and lower sections. The more oxygen gets in when we inhale, the better is the ventilation of our lungs, and more oxygen is absorbed and carried by our blood erythrocytes to produce energy. Thanks to this kind of breathing, children are robust, active, and happy.

Grown people breathe in an entirely different way. As we progress in years, lead an inactive lifestyle, suffer from spine misalignment, obesity etc., we start breathing differently. When we breathe in, our rib cage expands, our abdomen is deflated, our shoulders and collarbone move upwards. Only the upper, smallest sections of the lungs are involved in this kind of breathing. It usually does not provide enough air and we have to breathe more frequently (It is particularly noticeable in obese people.) Only small amounts of inhaled oxygen get into our lungs. The lungs work intensively but only in their upper parts. They become overworked and their cells suffer premature wear. There are layers of dead, inactive cells in the lung tissue.

The older we get the larger sections of our lungs are no longer involved in the breathing process. Our body is constantly oxygen-starved. This causes not only respiratory diseases but also disorders of circulatory system, pancreas, liver, kidneys, gastrointestinal tract, and many more.

We can delay our aging by thirty to forty years and avoid many diseases by utilizing the diaphragm better. It has been known for a long time that people of high longevity breathe slowly. A 130-year old East Indian person who looked half his age, when asked about the secret of his longevity said, "It is correct breathing" (he breathed once a minute). One of the principles of ancient medicine states: **"The fewer times we breathe in one minute, the longer our life is."**

Correct breathing is the assurance of good health and longevity. I reveal secrets of different breathing methods in the chapter "Breath of Life."

INCORRECT DIET

What we consume and what consumes us

Most families in a contemporary household consider three criteria when buying their food:

1. High in calories – that way we do not need to eat much of it.
2. Fast and easy to prepare – we are too busy with other things.
3. Easily absorbed without much chewing – modern people do not use their teeth much and do not have time for chewing.

Based on these criteria, meat seems to be better than vegetables because a small amount can satisfy our hunger. Pre-processed products are more in demand than the fresh ones because they do not require much work. Even store-bought juices are more often used than freshly squeezed ones. White bread and buns seem to be better than whole-grain products because they are easier to chew. Refined rice and sugar look very attractive. Our progressed society can arrange everything for our convenience. Even mothers do not need to worry about breastfeeding their babies. Baby formulas can substitute mother's milk. This kind of diet eventually harms even people with strong immune systems. Those with poor immunity start suffering much earlier. Children suffer the worst consequences of a poor diet.

The danger of refined foods

Sweet killer

Our desire to "improve" everything and to separate "needed" ingredients from the "unneeded" ones leads us to refining most of our food products. Our artificially "improved" food only seemingly has the same nutritious qualities as natural food. Artificial and natural foods have as little in common as silk roses with real ones – they only look similar. The same difference exists between synthetic and natural vitamins or synthetic margarine and real butter.

The objective of refining food is to make it more attractive commercially. Cooking and other forms of temperature treatment causes the food to lose its biological information (the total content and composition of chemical substances in natural products) acquired from the Sun, the Earth, and from water. Our body does not readily recognize and assimilate this sort of food. It has to draw from its own resources in order to make the food useful. Sugar beets, and sugar acquired from them, are a good example. Sugar beets are natural plant products containing many vitamins, mineral salts, enzymes, and hormones. On the contrary, sugar acquired from the beets is thoroughly refined, crystallized, and filtered. (A poison, calcium chloride, is used to make it white.) It gets into our stomach as a chemically pure substance, sucrose, without any vitamins, mineral salts, or other biologically active substances. Pure sucrose cannot be assimilated; it has to be joined with other substances. Beets have all the necessary substances in them; sugar does not. Our body is forced to use its own resources of calcium, iron, and other elements. This causes tooth decay, diabetes, anemia, etc. Research suggests that high consumption of sugar causes degeneration of blood vessels and individual cells, mutations, and eventually may lead to cancer.

We do not consume sugar only with our coffee and tea; it is in our candies, biscuits, cakes, and soft drinks. There are countless products containing sugar.

Because of high sugar consumption, the number of cases of diabetes, anemia, and blood cancers increased rapidly in the last twenty years in all developed countries. This is why parents and grandparents make a serious error when they treat children with candies and let them acquire a taste for sweets. The habit may be very difficult to eliminate later in the child's life.

Addiction to milk

Disease in a bottle

These days, it is common to substitute mother's milk with cow milk or baby formulas. **Human breast milk is rich in lactose that creates an environment that is favorable for the development of friendly bacteria in the baby's large intestine.**

Cow's milk contains certain types of proteins and antibodies, not possible for a baby to digest. These substances, instead of regular fermentation, undergo rotting in the baby's intestine, when the baby is fed with cow's milk or other substitutes. This causes autotoxication, imbalance in the microflora, and leads to the degeneration of the baby's intestine.

Substitutes do not have the biological information contained in mother's milk, and that causes the baby to constantly feel hungry and require frequent feeding. Because of that, starch and meat products are usually sooner included in the diet. The baby's digestive system is not fully formed; therefore it is not ready to digest and absorb these products. Certain necessary enzymes are not present in it. We can notice that many children, two to five years old, constantly have a mucous substance under their noses. It is caused by too much protein and starch in their diet. Artificial diet eventually destroys our children's immune system. They become vulnerable to all kinds of infections, such as frequent colds, runny nose, flu and pneumonia. Babies fed this way are, in most cases, allergy sufferers. We cannot predict all possible health problems caused by the absence of breast milk in our babies' diet.

Every future mother ought to know that nothing can substitute mother's breast milk; it is the natural food for her babies. No formula contains information about love, sensitivity, tenderness, or ways to avoid disasters and diseases. All this information comes from the mother and is encoded in her breast milk.

If a pregnant woman's diet consists mainly of sweets, white flour products, deli products, cow milk, coffee, fried or baked meat and other refined products, her child is going to suffer serious health consequences. It is even worse when she smokes cigarettes.

Who needs ulcers?

The content of iron in cow's milk is very low. Besides drinking its mother's milk, a calf also eats grass. Nature provided its digestive organs with the ability to separately digest milk and grass. Our digestive system is built differently. When cow's milk gets into our stomach, acidic digestive juices cause it to coagulate and form sticky matter similar to cheese. This "cheese" encloses pieces of other food in the stomach. The coagulated milk has to be digested before the other food. If this process occurs frequently, it can cause disorders of our digestive system, specifically ulceration of our stomach and duodenum. Do we really want our body to become a milk processing plant that brings us ulcers instead of expected benefits?

The main argument of milk drinking proponents is the high content of proteins (amino acids) and calcium in milk. I do not entirely agree with this argument and I will explain why.

Indigestible casein

No mammals in the world (except humans) consume milk when they are grown up. It would not be in accordance with nature. In the case of cats, we taught them to drink milk. However, it has been proven that cats live twice as long if they do not drink milk.

The difference between human milk and cow's milk is the high content of casein in the latter. Casein is a protein needed by the calf for building its hoofs and horns. A calf drinks its mother's milk only in the first six months of its life. Human beings do not have hoofs or horns. Why would they need so much casein?

Firstly, we do not need as much protein as most of us include in our diet. Our large intestine has a special kind of bacteria able to synthesize proteins from carbohydrates contained in plant-based foods (if the intestinal microflora is healthy).

Secondly, our body contains all elements found in Mendeleyev's table and all chemical compounds it needs, even though only 40% of them are supplied by the food we eat. Where do the compounds come from? They are synthesized in our body. It has a perfect chemical laboratory created by nature, with its capacity ranging from synthesizing amino acids to producing healing formulas, hormones, etc.

Let's go back to the synthesis of proteins. The air we inhale contains 80% more nitrogen (the main ingredient of amino acids) than the air we exhale. What happens with all that nitrogen? Our body uses it in the synthesis of amino acids. We can live eating very small amounts of animal proteins for a year, two years, or even longer without any danger to our health as long as we have air to breathe and eat enough vegetables and fruits. On the other hand, eating only proteins can result in our death in just one month. (In Shao Lin monastery people condemned to death were fed only meat and they died in twenty to forty days.)

When planning our diet, we ought to follow the proportions created by nature in woman's milk: a high content of simple car-

bohydrates and low protein content. Unfortunately, we do not always understand such hints given us by nature.

Casein contained in milk is broken down in the stomach by rennet. Children one to two years old already have hair and nails and do not need casein. Their digestive system does not produce rennet anymore, and casein becomes indigestible, even poisonous.

Undigested casein is the source of lumps in various parts of our body, forms kidney stones, clogs our blood vessels, and deforms our fingers. Other undigested cow milk ingredients build up in the form of mucous substances in our tissues and tendons.

Mucus is a substance swarming with disease-causing bacteria. Natural therapists believe that cow's milk is the source of mucous substances in our body throughout our entire life. This is why cow milk drinkers often make their body a host for bacteria that cause diseases such as flu, colds, asthma, bronchitis, and many others.

There is another fact worth mentioning. Today's milk is also harmful, especially for children, because of environmental pollution. Calcium in milk is always found together with radioactive strontium-90. Its molecular structure is similar to that of calcium but larger. When strontium-90 gets into our body, its molecules replace calcium molecules in our skeletal system. This is why milk drinkers have enlarged limbs (especially fingers and toes) and often suffer from hip and knee joints disorders.

Calcium, fat and cholesterol

There is no denying that milk is rich in calcium, the element necessary for the development of our bones. What about nuts, cabbage, carrots, beets or poppy seeds? In fact, they contain more calcium in an easily absorbable form, in an ideal proportion with other ingredients.

Milk also contains animal fat and, as we know, fat increases our levels of cholesterol (the main cause of heart diseases and circulatory problems). This is the main reason why milk is skimmed. However, the natural proportion of ingredients is destroyed in the process. Drinking such milk interferes with our body's ability to run its phosphorus-calcium economy in a balanced manner. Consequently, our ability to absorb calcium is decreased. Poor calcium absorption is one of the main causes of future osteoporosis. Skimming milk is supposed to save

23

our circulatory system (such is the common opinion I do not agree with) but it ruins our skeletal system. Are we really so addicted to milk that we are willing to risk our health?

Products such as plain yogurt, cheese, etc are different – they are safe to consume (in small quantities), even beneficial (especially if they have natural fat content). They are specifically recommended for the elderly and children. The bacteria found in those products perform most of the processing that our body would have to do at a great expenditure of its own resources – vitamins, mineral salts, macro-, and micro-elements.

Quitting the addiction

All these arguments are probably not going to persuade those for whom milk and dairy products are the main part of their diet. It is not easy to quit a life-long addiction. If you cannot quit drinking milk, at least switch to goat milk. It is low in casein and fat, and resembles human milk in its content.

If you continue drinking cow's milk, watch for such symptoms as intestinal pains, bloating, diarrhea, constipation, increased pain in bones and joints, etc. "To drink or not to drink?" – that is your own decision.

The truth about meat – the time bomb

I would like to say a few words about meat – the product I do not recommend for everyday consumption. Consuming large amounts of animal proteins (meat, deli etc.), in amounts exceeding our body's daily demand, causes rotting processes, constipation, and poisoning of the body by lactic, oxalic, and uric acids (the three main culprits responsible for joint diseases, back pain, osteoporosis, and other mobility-reducing disorders).

Meat itself does not have taste nor smell so we fry, cook, and season it to improve its taste. When meat is processed, it releases about 20 poisonous substances that can cause damage to blood vessels and the nervous system. The digestion of meat requires large amounts of vitamins and microelements. **If we do not eat adequate amounts of** raw vegetable salads together with meat, digestion is incomplete and the undigested meat putrefies in our intestines. The putrefaction processes increase the alkalinity of our large intestine, which leads to blood acidity. Alkaline environment promotes the development of diseased cells (especially cancerous). Those who excessively consume meat are the prime candidates for cancer.

There is one more fact that requires your attention. **Excessive consumption of animal proteins, especially in early childhood, puts us at risk of immune system disorders. The digestion of meat needs large amounts of vitamins and microelements that are taken from the child's blood. Depleted levels of these substances cause the development of hidden anemia and blood diseases. Ironically, all kinds of allergies, eczemas, and other disorders typical for the age of puberty are usually the result of our parents' well-intended care. Unaware of the dangers, they cause damage to their children's health by including too much meat in the diet.**

Eastern philosophy teaches that each food product we consume contains information about its place of birth and development: - the climate, the exposure to sunrays, moonlight, etc. What kind of information can be contained in meat? Times when cattle were grazing on green pastures are long over. They are raised their entire lives without sunlight or fresh air. Instead of eating fresh, juicy grass, they are fed hormones and various synthetic feeds.

When we buy a shapeless piece of meat, we do not think that it was once a part of a lovable animal that was killed by electrocution. It is naive to believe that animals do not sense impending death in their last moments. They sense it very clearly. Faced with aggression and driven by fear, a slaughtered animal's body produces large amounts of poisonous hormones, which we consume later as we enjoy our steaks. No wonder that both adults and children become increasingly aggressive and hot-tempered. Aggression always breeds aggression - this old truth is confirmed by the results of high meat consumption.

In recent years (1999-2002), the number of BSE (Mad Cow Disease) cases in Western Europe has grown to epidemic proportions. Cattle affected by BSE experience a complete degeneration of their nervous system (sections of their brain tissue turn spongy). Instead of feeding cattle exclusively with plant-based food, the industry started using animal proteins in the form of meat and bone meal. BSE is a vivid example of physiological changes that can be caused by eating improper food. To prevent the spread of BSE, whole herds of cattle are slaughtered and incinerated. May God prevent children whose diet is based on meat from the consequences of unnatural feeding practices in the cattle industry!

Less flour – more power

Refined flour makes us suffer

Let's take a look at flour – a common product in our households. It is made from grains. Unrefined flour contains vitamins B, PP, and F, mineral salts, enzymes, and other ingredients needed in our body. A grain consists of 85% starch and 15% biological coating. The substances contained in the coating allow us to break down and absorb the starch.

Refined flour does not have the coating – it is poor in vitamins, enzymes and minerals.

The digestion of white bread or buns requires a number of substances that are removed in the refining process. Our digestive system is going to take them from our body's resources. Refined flour is hard to digest. Undigested starch remains in the fat layers of our body. We know what happens to flour when it is mixed with warm water. It expands and forms a glue-like substance. Refined flour behaves the same way in our intestines, slowing the digestion of other foods and forming gallstones or bladder stones.

We add substances such as food coloring, aromas, acidity modifiers, stabilizers, and thickeners in order to make our breads, buns, cakes, biscuits, and other refined flour products more attractive. What happens with these additives? They remain in the body and gradually poison us. They cause our muscles and joints to stiffen. This is how white flour products can cause us a lot of suffering.

The danger of yeast

The production of practically all types of bread involves the use of yeast. When we bake, yeast spores constantly float in the air and land on the bread's surface. The spores travel with bread to our digestive tract, where they become active. There has been some American research showing that baker's yeast activates cancerous cells in our body. When we eat leavened bread, we turn our digestive tract into a "battle-field" between yeast and our natural intestinal microflora. Since we start eating bread in our childhood, a healthy intestinal microflora is a rarity.

Constipation, bloating, and digestive tract diseases are often effects of consuming large amounts of bread and various other baked goods made from refined flour with the use of baker's yeast.

Unleavened bread
(made solely from wheat flour and water, without yeast)

Leavened bread was invented in Egypt about 15 thousand years ago, and its negative effects have been known for a long time. Many nations, in order to preserve their populations, avoided leavened bread, and they recorded this custom in the form of religious commandments. For example in the Bible (Ex.12), we read: "Nothing leavened may you eat; wherever you dwell you may eat only unleavened bread." It is very wise and useful advice. The idea of giving up raised white bread and buns may be shocking for some people but, if you value your health, you should consider taking that step.

You are better off eating bread made of unrefined flour without the use of yeast.

If you continue eating leavened bread, do not eat it fresh – after one to two days yeast is not active or harmful anymore. You can make it more attractive by toasting it, making biscuits, etc.

The vicious circle

All refined grains lose valuable substances contained in their coating and become pure starch that is hard to absorb. Unrefined grain products are much better for our health. In general, refined foods such as deli products, chips, baked goods etc., usually contain not enough water and too much sugar or salt. We usually have to follow them by a drink to quench our thirst. **This creates a vicious circle: Refined food stimulates our thirst, we drink more fluids, they dilute digestive juices in our stomach, and digestion is incomplete. Salt irritates**

27

our stomach so we drink more to neutralize it. This way we eat and drink almost continuously. Consequently, we fill our bodies with fluids, gain weight and feel tired.

Our diet and our mood

The Japanese like to joke: "If a couple starts their day with a fight, they should recall what they ate the previous day." As this simple saying points out refined products damage not only our physical health but also influence our mind. Some American psychologists believe that by reducing sugar, meat and coffee in our diet we can reduce aggressive behavior by 50%. Our ancestors realized the importance of that fact much earlier. There is a saying in the East: "God created food and the devil created a chef." One could ask: "How can I live without meat, white bread and buns, coffee, sweets, chocolate, etc.?" Use your imagination! There are a great variety of foods provided by nature. When you crave a lot, you can still have a candy, a piece of your favorite cake, or a slice of smoked meat – but you have to remember that they are poisons!

We are what we eat

The health of your digestive tract, from your teeth to your large intestine, depends largely on your understanding of the following information.

Let's look at our typical sandwich – usually including bread or a bun, butter, and some kind of deli meat - followed by a drink of pop, coffee or tea. Bread is classified as carbohydrate food, butter belongs to fats, and meat belongs to the protein food group. The combination of these products forms in our stomach a mixture that is hard to digest.

Carbohydrates are digested in our mouth and partially in the duodenum while proteins in our stomach and duodenum. Different digestive juices are produced for that purpose and they need different amounts of time to perform their functions. When butter gets into our stomach, the action of those juices is suppressed. The digestive process slows down and food remains in the stomach for a long time. When we follow it by a drink (pop, coffee, tea), we wash undigested food and acidic digestive juice from our stomach to the duodenum. The duodenum has an alkaline environment. The acidic diges-

tive juice damages the mucous lining in the duodenum and causes its inflammation and, with time, ulceration. **Then the undigested remains of food reach the large intestine where undigested bread causes rotting processes and the deli products become stagnant fecal matter.** We will soon find out how those deposits affect our health.

Some people cannot imagine life without sandwiches. I am not against sandwiches as such. We can eat sandwiches consisting of bread, butter, and some tomato or cucumber. We can also enjoy a slice of cheese or smoked meat wrapped in lettuce. **However, a sandwich made of bread, butter, and some kind of deli meat product is a combination most harmful for our digestive tract**. It is an example of incorrect combinations of food products that can damage your health.

From what kind of food should we get our life energy? The kind that grows in the sunlight is the best source of energy for us. The sun is the universal energy source for every living organism. Nature gave plants the ability to absorb and accumulate sun energy that is later available for our use.

Nutrition influences not only our health but also our longevity. We know how to calculate calories we consume in a day. Our daily mixed diet (including ice cream, candy, coffee etc.) gives us about 2,500 kcal. According to scientific calculations, an average person uses up about 50,000,000 kcal in the lifetime. Based on it, let's try to calculate the average lifetime (assuming mixed diet). If we divide 50,000,000 kcal (lifetime use) by 2,500 kcal (daily use), we get 20,000 days or 55 years.

Now try to calculate what should be the average lifetime of those who eat natural products and use about 1,000 kcal a day: 50,000,000 kcal / 1,000 kcal a day gives us 50,000 days or 137 years. It is not just arithmetic anymore; we are talking about our life.

It is a scientific fact that there is one vegetarian for 1,000 meat eaters in the age group under sixty; in the seventy-and-over group, the proportion is 100 to 1,000; over the age of eighty, there are 600 vegetarians for 1,000 meat-eaters.

I would like to add that diet based only on the calorie count is wrong from the physiological point of view. It is not the initial calorie content of the food that matters, but how much energy we actually obtain from it when it is digested.

Even though plant-based foods represent lower calorie content, net energy our body receives after their digestion is still higher. This is why a bowl of buckwheat makes us feel light and ready to do some work. In contrast, eating a portion of meat makes us feel like having a cup of coffee and going to sleep. Many people associate meat consumption with strength and energy. In reality, meat only stimulates our nervous system in a similar way narcotics do.

The important thing in our food is the balance of ingredients: proteins, carbohydrates, fats, minerals, vitamins, and microelements. If their amounts are properly balanced (as they are in natural foods), our body uses only small amounts of energy for digestion. Most energy can be used for cleaning up toxins and making repairs. All artificial foods lack the perfect balance of ingredients. Their digestion becomes a very complex task and uses up all energy contained in those products. In some cases digestion requires more energy than the food contains. It takes large amounts of such foods to kill hunger. On one hand, we try to control the number of meals we eat; on the other hand, we still have to deal with obesity. We put unnecessary stress on our body by trying weight-reduction programs and remedies. The programs end and obesity comes back.

The conclusion is: No program, diet, or chef can balance the amounts of proteins, fat, carbohydrates, vitamins, and microelements in our meals the same way they are balanced in plant-based products.

Not everybody has to be a vegetarian

I do not want to be misunderstood – not everybody has to become a vegetarian. I am not trying to convince you to stay away from all earthly pleasures and blessings that give life half of its charm. We can have feasts in our life when we are allowed to eat all kinds of foods, but on ordinary days we should stick to what is healthy for our body.

Use moderation in eating because it is one of the basic conditions of our survival.

Illness on a plate

A commission of the World Health Organization did some research in a few Tibetan monasteries. It turned out that the monks were physically fit and almost completely healthy. There was no tooth decay, circulatory disorders or digestive disorders in 60% of the cases. Their

30

diet is very modest. They do not have refrigerators or natural gas stoves; they never eat meat, sugar or any refined product. The main items on their menu are barley cakes, herbal tea and clear water. Turnips, carrots, and rice enrich the diet in the summertime.

Ironically, in such developed countries as the USA, Germany or France, where the consumption of milk, meat, refined products, and wider selection of food types is the greatest, the general health level is poor.

In the USA, for example, two families out of three have been touched by cancer, two people out of five suffer and die from heart problems, and many suffer from diabetes. Chronic diseases affect 19% of the population – close to one out of five people.

In Germany 20% of the population suffers from diabetes and 20% of the children age eight to sixteen have developmental problems, both physical and intellectual. Rheumatism and joint inflammations affect 15-17% of the people.

In France 15-20% of the people have allergies. There are 450 thousand children under 18 with hearing and sight problems, and 1.5 million children aged six and under suffer from asthma. In all highly industrialized countries the number of children born with some kind of health disorder doubled in the last 25 years.

An old Tibetan adage teaches: **"Most people get ill for one of two reasons – overeating or hunger." As it turns out, we often use forks and spoons to dig our own graves.**

The knowledge allowing us to use a correct diet is very important. It is not enough to prepare tasty meals; we need to know how to properly nurture our bodies.

In the chapter "Food", page 101, you can find answers to questions about combining products correctly to enhance your health.

LACK OF INTERNAL BODY HYGIENE

Look after your health as carefully and tenderly as you look after your car

We hear from our childhood about external body hygiene, but we know little about internal hygiene. However, the condition

of our internal organs determines much of our external appearance.

Each owner keeps his car clean inside and outside. Best quality oil and fuel are used. Why don't we care for our health with an equal sense of responsibility? If we don't clean the inside of our car for a year, there will be plenty of dirt and dust. Most people never clean the inside of their body. Usually around the age of forty, their body is so tired of poisons, harmful deposits, and unfriendly bacteria that it becomes susceptible to disease.

Our body is built of cells. Nature created us in such a way that every second as many new cells are built as many old ones die. In a constantly poisoned body, there are more old cells than new ones. This kind of unhealthy imbalance causes disease and the degeneration of our body as we age.

The evolution began from a simple single-cell organism with two openings: one for taking food in and one for discharging waste. All life processes happen between those two openings. If the process of waste discharge malfunctions, the cell dies. It is a simple but perfect model. Our body contains billions of cells but the general principle is still the same: a malfunctioning waste discharge system causes diseases and death.

Not many of us know that a grown person's large intestine contains 17-33 lb (8-15 kg) of hardened fecal material that we carry around all life long.

Usually after the age of 40, our large intestine is so full of fecal matter that it crowds out other organs and interferes with the functioning of our liver, kidneys, and lungs. It is a considerable cause of many diseases. Let me explain how it works.

All food products are commonly divided into four groups:

1. Proteins – meat, fish, eggs etc.
2. Carbohydrates – bread, honey, candy, potatoes etc.
3. Fats – butter, oil, grease etc.
4. Fruits and vegetables, fruit juices

The digestion of most of carbohydrates, fruits and vegetables starts in the mouth and continues in the small intestine. Fats and proteins are digested in the stomach.

Eating meat and potatoes together is enough to cause digestive problems. We do not think about different digestion times for different food products. However the digestion of potatoes takes about one hour; meat needs three to seven hours to be digested.

A lot of our body's energy that can be used for life processes and fighting disease is wasted on digestion and disposing waste from a dinner consisting of incorrectly combined food products. Remains of undigested food get into our large intestine, separate from digested food, and form layers of stagnant fecal matter.

Our large intestine is like a pot containing fertile soil in the form of digested food. The body is like a plant. The walls of the large intestine are lined with roots that, like roots of a plant, absorb nutritious substances into our blood. Each group of roots nurtures a specific organ. Useless waste is discarded. What happens with the undigested chunk?

During the next meal, a new chunk sticks to the old one, then another one. Undigested food sticks to the large intestine's walls. We carry around with us a few pounds of those chunks. It is not hard to imagine what happens with food products "stored" for many years in temperatures above 97F (36C).

The intestine still performs its absorbing function under this layer of filth and delivers toxins, carcinogenic substances - products of decay, to the body. Obviously, this is not a good material for building healthy cells. The toxins circulate with blood and gradually ruin our health.

We can conclude from the above that we can never have only a single diseased organ. The entire body is ill. One organ gives in first but treating it does not solve the problem. When we treat a specific illness, we treat the local symptom of a bigger underlying problem – the pollution of the whole body. While we treat a specific disorder, the main culprit remains untreated and is ready to strike anywhere. The poisoned intestine is constantly delivering toxic substances to the entire body. It becomes the source of general poisoning. Deposits of stagnant fecal matter form hardened layers. The huge sack of waste pushes internal organs out of their proper places, creates pressure on the diaphragm, and eliminates it from the breathing process, lowering significantly the capacity of our lungs. The liver is pushed out of its place; there is pressure on the kidneys; the small intestine does not have enough space for its movements; men find their genital-urinary systems crowded. The lower section of the rectum is put under most stress; overworked veins expand and form bloody lumps. A poisoned large intestine can cause countless problems and diagnosis of diseases is unpredictable. In the worst-case scenario, last stages of cancer, the passage of waste in the large intestine is completely blocked and the body dies poisoned by its own toxins (autotoxication).

Autotoxication

Self-poisoning (autotoxication) is the worst enemy of our health. It is the cause of many diseases because all of them begin in poisoned blood.

Ancient physicians and healers of Egypt and Tibet knew long ago the fundamental principle: **Good health requires maintaining our intestines in perfect order.**

"Many diseases enter our body through the mouth," said **Hippocrates.** As usual, he was right.

We tend to eat many cooked and flour-based products combined with butter and sugar along with proteins (meat, deli products, cheese, dairy, eggs). Because our digestive system is not able to completely process meals containing a variety of different foods mixed together, the walls of our large intestine become lined with chunks of undigested food. The large intestine's environment is warm and humid. Remains of undigested food become a mass full of unfriendly bacteria; they produce toxins – poisonous byproducts of their own metabolism. The walls of our large intestine absorb these toxins; they circulate with blood and gradually poison our body.

As we can see, overeating and improper combining of food products cause most damage to our gastrointestinal tract.

Unusual coloring of the tongue, bad breath, sudden headaches, dizziness, apathy, sleepiness, heaviness in the lower abdomen, and bloating can all be results of autotoxication caused by constipation.

The absence of bowel movement for more than 24 hours is an obvious case of constipation and definitely requires a remedy.

It is no secret that 60% of people suffer from chronic constipation. Let's point out the main reasons for such unhealthy condition of most people's large intestine.

1. Consuming food rich in calories and low in volume. We often kill hunger by having a sandwich followed by a drink of pop, tea, or coffee. Due to its small volume, the sandwich produces little fecal material in the large intestine and does not create enough pressure on the bowels to cause defecation. We might not feel any need for bowel movement for a few days.

2. Consuming excessive volumes of food. It has been known for a long time that people eat three to five times as much as it is necessary for their bodies. When we overeat, not all food can be absorbed and some of it starts rotting. Our intestines become a battlefield between the friendly bacteria and the disease-causing bacteria. The discharge of waste is suspended until this battle is over.

3. Consuming large amounts of coffee and flour-based products (bread, pastry, etc.) without enough products rich in fiber that would make our large intestine work.

Blood means life

Our body is built of cells, cells form tissues, and tissues build organs. Organs are parts of organ systems (nervous, skeletal, etc.) and all systems are closely interconnected. The cells get nutrients from blood. Blood sustains life as long as it is saturated with energy, microelements, hormones, and vitamins. Only blood free of poisons can build healthy cells, bones, skin, hair, and teeth. **Blood polluted with toxins caused by frequent constipation becomes the source of self-poisoning.**

According to some statistics, in nine cases out of ten, women with breast cancer have observably slower intestine function. Had they had preventative procedures (the cleaning of their large intestine) done 10-15 years earlier, they probably would have never gotten breast cancer or any other kind of cancer.

The microflora of the large intestine

There are over 500 kinds of bacteria in our large intestine. **In a healthy intestine these bacteria complete the digestion of food and destroy other, disease causing, bacteria. They also produce essential vitamins, hormones, enzymes, and amino acids.** Eating large amounts of animal proteins causes constant putrefaction processes in our large intestine and results in emission of methane. This poisonous gas destroys bacteria that produce B vitamins and prevent our body from producing cancerous cells. As we can see, the absence of only one kind of bacteria can cause countless complications to our health.

Large intestine – the "fuse" of our health

Nature provided us with a robust immune system. The large intestine is an important part of it. Each segment of the intestine stimulates a specific organ in our body. If our large intestine is healthy, no diseases can threaten us. However, if there are unhealthy deposits in our intestine, or its microflora is out of balance, our health is in danger. On the picture, we can see possible diseases caused by deposits in our large intestine.

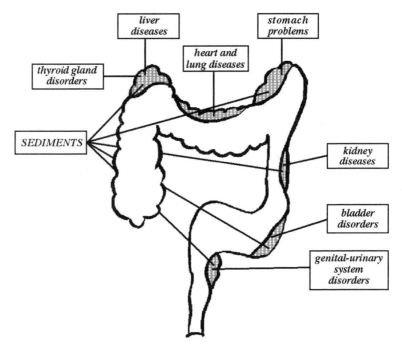

Fig. 1. Diseases caused by unhealthy deposits in the large intestine.

Here are some external symptoms of unhealthy large intestine:

1. Bloating, constipation, gas
2. Black stains on the teeth
3. Grey, white, or yellowish color of the tongue
4. Warts and freckles on the skin

Seven cleaning systems in our body

There are seven systems responsible for cleaning mucus, tars, and other filth out of our body. These systems are:

1. The large intestine
2. The liver
3. The kidneys
4. Fat tissue
5. Muscles and tendons
6. Nose, ears, and eyes
7. Lungs and skin

When one of our internal cleaning systems is not able to do its job, the next system is turned on. For example, if the large intestine and liver cannot complete the cleaning tasks, the systems connected with the nose, eyes, skin, and lungs take over. The result is rashes, eczema, allergies, runny nose, phlegm coughed up from the lungs from time to time, and secretion from the eyes.

In such cases, people use nose drops, put compresses on their eyes, or rub medicated creams onto their skin. All these measures only fight the symptoms. The treatment is usually long, costly, and ineffective.

"Each illness has its cause, and the cause cannot be removed by any medication".

— Hippocrates

The medication or hospital care cannot cure us from bad habits that result in the internal contamination of our body.

If we closely examined our internal cleaning systems, we would find out that in most cases they are in a terrible condition:

- The large intestine is so contaminated that our blood absorbs more filth than useful substances from it.

37

- The liver or gallbladder are so plugged with stones, cholesterol, and dark-green bile that the process of filtering toxins out of blood is suppressed.
- The kidneys are not able to do their function because they are stuffed with sand and stones.
- Salty deposits on the bones and joints cause pain with every movement of the neck, arms, or knees. The joints produce a crunching sound when they return to their resting position.

How can we expect to feel healthy with so much internal contamination in our body?

Our body's ability to complete the cleansing task on its own depends on the level of contamination.

The levels of internal body contamination

First – The constant feeling of fatigue despite a healthy body appearance
Second – Headaches and bone pains
Third – Many types of allergies
Forth – Cysts, lumps, stones, and obesity
Fifth – Deformed internal organs, bones, and joints
Sixth – Nervous system diseases
Seventh – The degeneration of cells and organs, eventually leading to cancers

You can determine the level of your body's internal contamination by watching the symptoms. If you notice symptoms of the second and third level, you do not have much time to waste – start the procedure of complete body cleansing as soon as possible.

Can we be proud of our human ways?

If we wanted to live by nature's laws, we would use the blessings of sunlight, air, water, and land. We got used to processed foods, which have to be sweet, tasty, cooked, and warm. This is why our body cannot live and function to its full potential.

No pills are going to cure us when our blood is contaminated with poisons. Diseases cause permanent damage to our health, our heart becomes weak, and our brain dies. We have two choices: put up with the illness and expect a premature death or clean up our body's "dirty swamp" and adopt a healthy lifestyle.

In the chapter "Complete Body Cleansing" you can find a method that suits you best for keeping your gastrointestinal tract in good order and choose a therapy for removing toxins and other harmful deposits accumulated in your body over the years.

INABILITY TO LIVE A BLISSFUL LIFE

It is important to understand that each disorder in our body has not only physical but also psychological causes.

Our way of thinking influences what happens to us and determines good and bad aspects of our life. Listen to your own words. If you notice that you express the same thought repeatedly, a few days in a row, it has become your mental template. We all live by our thoughts – they direct our actions. **If our thoughts are full of anger, fear, pain, sadness, and vengeance, what kinds of actions can they result in? If our thoughts are positive, we can usually expect all the best in our life but negative thinking can only bring difficulties and failure.**

It appears that our way of thinking not only determines our life's successes and failures but also has a vital influence on our health. For example, many people suffer from headaches, neck pains, and back pains. What could be the cause of these pains? Our neck can be mentally associated with flexibility. In our thoughts and actions, flexibility means the ability to approach a problem from different points of view and creativity in finding a solution. People who are stubborn, unable to compromise, and cannot see the problem from their opponent's point of view will suffer from headaches, neck pains and back pains until they learn to treat somebody else's opinion with greater compassion and understanding. If we habitually criticize everybody and everything, our joints and muscles start hurting. When anger and hatred dominate our thoughts, our body "burns out" and is susceptible to infections. If we keep dwelling on some injustice we suffered long time ago, it "consumes" our body and eventually leads to the creation of cancerous cells and then cancers.

39

We should work on eliminating negative thoughts and stereotypes as early as possible to achieve not only psychological but also physical health. It is a very difficult art to learn, and we all have to learn it on our own.

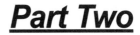
Part Two

HEALTHY SPINE
— THE FOUNDATION
OF A HEALTHY BODY

Most people's spines are so degenerated that it takes a lot of time and patience to correct the maladjustments. Pain does not go away as fast as we would wish.

Nevertheless, everything can be corrected. **We should acquire the habit of looking after our health, and understand that we are the custodians of our bodies. To keep our spine strong and healthy, we should sleep on a firm mattress, use a firm pillow, and follow a daily exercise routine.**

Why is sleeping on a firm mattress beneficial to our health?

We sleep about one third of our lifetime. When we sleep, our muscles relax and our body stretches. All our movements are different from the movements we do when we are awake. Movements in our sleep require less energy – sleep is the best time for our spine's rehabilitation.

The mattress we sleep on should be as firm as possible without disturbing our sleep. We should sleep in a straight position, on our backs, with our arms stretched alongside the body and our legs relaxed. In such position, our weight is distributed evenly, our muscles are very relaxed, and all dislocations of vertebrae, we might have encountered during the day, are slightly corrected.

The heart works under little strain in this position, easily pumping the blood, and the circulation is good. Better blood circulation means easier work for our liver as it removes toxins from our body.

A well functioning liver means better metabolism. That way we can lose six to ten pounds (three to five kilograms) of weight, and get rid of many health problems after just two months of sleeping on a firm mattress.

In the first few days of sleeping on a firm mattress, we will feel muscle and spine pain. When the misalignment of vertebrae is corrected (10-14 days), the pain will disappear.

Why is sleeping on a soft mattress harmful?

Our liver is the chemical laboratory of our body. Thousands of chemical reactions, collectively known as metabolism, depend on the proper functioning of this laboratory.

43

Science shows that even spacing of the thoracic vertebrae, starting from the third up to the twentieth, allows efficient functioning of the liver. People who sleep on soft mattresses always have those vertebrae bowed, and that significantly worsens their liver's function.

The quality (firmness) of our mattress has a huge influence on our spine's condition and, indirectly, on our general health.

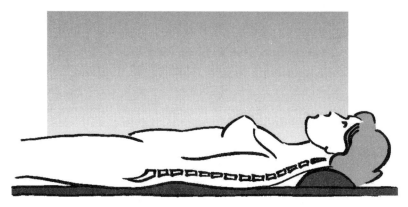

Fig. 2. Vertebrae are correctly positioned on a firm mattress and a small pillow.

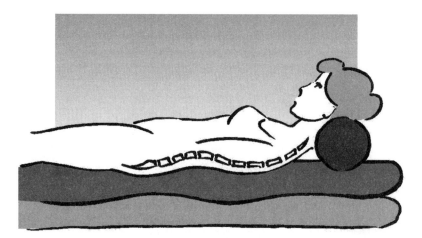

Fig. 3. Our spine is bent and becomes degenerated when we sleep on a soft mattress and a high pillow.

The above picture shows how a firm mattress can influence the condition of our spine. It is worthwhile to give some appreciation to the place where we spend a large part of our life. Our bed should serve our health well, rather than cause us strain and damage.

Why is a firm pillow good for our health?

The pillow we sleep on should be firm, small, and low. People who can sleep without a pillow should put a rolled up towel under their necks. A firm pillow helps maintain the nasal septum (partition) in good condition.

Our nasal septum is responsible for the physiological balance in the functioning of all our body organs. Easy breathing through both sides of our nose is very important for the proper functioning of our body. Beside that, air is warmed up, cleaned and disinfected when it passes through the nose.

When we sleep on soft, large, and high pillows, our spine is so bent that breathing through the nose becomes difficult and we start breathing through the mouth. This is dangerous for our health because all kinds of germs can easily get this way into our air passages.

Frequent colds, throat diseases, and bronchi problems are effects of sleeping on soft and high pillows.

A spine operation should be the last resort

People who are ill often consider an operation to be a panacea for all their disorders. There are about 200,000 different corrective procedures performed for lower back pain in the USA each year. Half of them do not bring any improvement and are not necessary in the first place.

The damaged disk is usually removed in a procedure. However, this may cause the necessity of another operation and the removal of another disk resulting in a stiff spine segment. Such an operation removes the immediate cause of stress on our nerve structures but does not remove the original cause of disk damage. An operation should be the last resort, when the preventative methods become ineffective.

We "earn" the good condition of our spine throughout our life. If

45

we habitually neglect our spine, we can expect that, sooner or later, we will have to deal with hard to tolerate pain. Then we will find time, even a lot of time, for therapy. Is it not better to spend some time and effort in order to prevent the problem?

Prevention is the best strategy to avoid spine problems

1. We should watch ourselves to make sure we walk, stand, and sit straight, pull our abdomen in, keep our back straight, and our head slightly raised.
2. We should never cross our legs while we sit because two large arteries run under our knees, and pressure on them interferes with the blood circulation, which with time causes spine and back pain, varicose veins, and problems with blood vessels in our lower limbs.
3. When we lift anything, we should not keep our knees straight. Bending them reduces strain on the spine.
4. Firm abdominal muscles reduce strain on our spine by 20%.
5. When we carry heavy items (for example groceries), we should distribute loads evenly on both shoulders

I suggest two sets of exercises for keeping a good posture and eliminating spinal pain. They do not require much time or effort and bring excellent results.

Exercise set number 1

– When you wake up, stretch a few times.
– Lying on your back, press hard against the pillow with the back of your head for 5 seconds and then rest for 5 seconds. Repeat the exercise 6 times.
– Put the pillow on your chest and "hug" it for 5 seconds – rest for 5 seconds. Repeat the exercise 6 times.
– Put the pillow between your knees and squeeze it hard for 5 seconds – rest for 5 seconds; repeat 6 times.
– Pull up your knees to the 45 degree angle – hold for 5 seconds and rest for 5 seconds; repeat 6 times.

– Pull the toes of one leg with the toes of the other leg towards you, alternately, six times for each leg.

Exercises done in bed put very little strain on our heart, therefore they can be done by anybody – children, adults, or elderly people.

Exercise set number 2

This set of exercises corrects the actions of our muscles, nerves, internal organs, and blood vessels; regulates the functioning of our nervous and digestive systems, and has good influence on our mental capabilities. I recommend it for people who lead active lifestyles and work intensively.

1. Sit down on a chair, move your feet slightly forward, put your hands on your knees, raise and then rest your arms 10 times.
2. In the same position, move your head alternately left and right 10 times each way.
3. Move your head back and forth – 10 times each way.
4. Stretch out your arms horizontally in front of you and turn your head alternately left and right 5 times each way.
5. Raise your arms at the 90-degree angle, push them back and at the same time move your chin forward and up. Repeat 10 times.

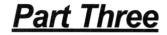
Part Three

OBESITY
— YOUR WORST ENEMY

Today I received again a stack of letters from my readers in the mail. I am grateful for the positive feedback about my work and the testimony of successful therapies based on my advice.

I would like to apologize for not providing an individual reply to each letter. There are many reasons for that – the main one is simply time constraints. Many answers can be found in my books. Please read them with due attention and try to comprehend the concepts. This book provides answers for some letters (see Questions and Answers, page 153). Please pay attention to the following letter dealing with a problem concerning many people.

> *I have been fighting obesity all my life. Whatever I have tried – diets, fasting, and slimming formulas – proved ineffective. I do not overeat and do not know where the fat comes from. Something may be wrong with my metabolism. Please tell me if you know any miracle diet. It is very important to me.* **Henryka M**

The fact that you are not alone with your problem should provide some comfort – 70% of Earth's population is overweight. This does not mean that I encourage you to give up. Let us analyze a number of obesity causes in modern people. Maybe this analysis can provide an answer to your and other people's concerns.

It may surprise many people to learn that there is a connection between obesity and the condition of the spine. Imagine that you are constantly burdened with 44lb (20 kg) extra weight every day and night. Would that affect your spine?

Based on many years of studying obesity cases, I personally concluded that there is a close connection between obesity and bad condition of the spine.

The spine controls our metabolism

The thirty-three vertebrae of our spine, besides keeping our body in a vertical position, have other important functions. We all know that they also provide support for the spinal cord and its nerve pathways used for directing the work of our internal organs. Lumbar vertebrae are of most interest to us because they enclose the section of the spinal cord that is responsible for regulating our metabolism. In other words, **if** our lumbar spine suffers degeneration (pathology) such as dislocation of vertebrae, we have the tendency to a fast weight gain or weight loss. This suggests a simple explanation for the fact that some people who do not eat much gain weight, while others are unusually slim despite overeating. Both groups have pathological changes in their lumbar vertebrae.

Abnormal body weight is caused by the degeneration of lumbar vertebrae that interferes with the transmission of nerve impulses to the internal organs, which in turn disturbs their normal functioning. This phenomenon is commonly described as metabolic disorders. The process of weight change is more dramatic in cases of more severe degeneration of the lumbar spine.

You may ask: "How can a degenerated spine be corrected?" I suggest learning about other causes of abnormal weight first, and considering corrective steps later.

Direct causes of obesity (hormonal disorders, improper processing of fats and carbohydrates) often originate in a degenerated lumbar spine. This is why no diet can, in the long run, stop abnormal weight gain or loss. Low-calorie diets, limiting the number of meals, or slimming formulas do not remove the causes of abnormal weight – they only fight the symptoms.

There are a few remarks I would like to make about dieting. Using diets over a long period is very dangerous for our circulatory system. Our body builds about 6.2 miles (10,000m) of blood vessels for servicing 2.2 lb (1kg) of fat tissue. If our weight changes frequently (from dieting), there is a constant stress on the circulatory system, resulting in serious wear of blood vessels and veins. Most people who constantly experiment with different diets have visibly swollen veins (mostly in their legs) or broken blood vessels under their skin.

In conclusion, limiting food intake alone can reduce body weight for some time, but it is also sure to damage the overall health and can lead to anemia, depressive states, and even worse - degeneration of the circulatory system.

Why are diet programs ineffective?

Most people who struggle with obesity choose one of the three methods:

1. Slimming formulas
2. Low calorie diets
3. Physical exercise

Let's analyze each of these methods.

1. **Slimming formulas.** Various weight-reducing pharmaceutical formulas are recently very popular. These formulas only bring temporary weight-reducing effects. In most cases, the positive effects disappear two to three months after quitting the formula. What is left is indescribable damage to our body, especially our liver, stomach, pancreas, and circulatory system. The formulas cause dehydration in our body, change the composition of our blood and make it thicker, increase our body's acidity (harmful!), etc. – the negative effects are not fully predictable. The therapies rely on artificial formulas to do the job without any psychological involvement of the patient. Our individuality deserves more appreciation – our bodies are different from one another and they have certain unique features.

This is why we all have to find an individual method to keep our body in a healthy shape; a method based on our body's unique physiology and not on mass-marketed formulas. The process of losing excess weight ought to be directed by our own mind. We want to lose excess pounds in order to improve our health, not to open the door for illness.

2. **Low calorie diets.** As we know, water is the base of fat tissue accumulating in our body. Any diet program or weight-reducing formula triggers our body's defense mechanisms: when it does not get enough nutrition, it has to use its own fat as an energy source for physiological processes. Water is a by-product of processing fat and is discarded by our body. Instead of slimming down, our body starts to dry up and resemble a dried fruit. The skin on our face and body becomes wrinkled; our muscles get flabby; we suffer from headaches, liver pains, and abdominal pains. Finally, the constant sensation of intense hunger and the feeling of weakness force us to break the diet. Fat tissue acts like a sponge ready to absorb water. The return to obesity can be very fast.

3. **Physical exercise.** Physical strain involved in exercise such as aerobic, jogging, etc., can lead an unprepared body to serious health

problems. This happens because intense physical exercise increases blood circulation and warms up our body. Harmful deposits accumulated inside our body in such places as intestines and blood vessels (obese people usually have larger harmful deposits) become more acidic and the amount of toxic substances increases. Heavy sweating removes some of the toxins, but our blood absorbs the bulk of them and circulates them in the body, causing autotoxication (self-poisoning). Our general health deteriorates, with acute headaches and depression as the first symptoms. In particular, people over thirty years of age should never try to reduce excess weight by intense physical exercise.

Obese people trying to lose weight by using one of the methods mentioned above make two fundamental mistakes:

> ***First***   – Dieting for only a period of time during which only low-calorie foods are consumed. (In fact, the word "diet" means in Greek "lifestyle", not a period of time.)
>
> ***Second*** – Trying to lose as many pounds as possible in a short time

An Eastern adage says: "You cannot have a baby born in one month by putting nine pregnant women together." To apply this simple truth to our discussion, there is no quick way – if we have been gaining weight for some years, it has to take time (two to three months) to turn this process around and set our body on the weight-reduction course.

One of the fundamental principles of nature states that nothing disappears without a trace and nothing comes to existence out of nothing. **This principle contains the most important lesson for the obese – eat less.**

Here is some advice on how to do it:

- Use smaller plates – half the size of plates you are using now.
- Learn to eat slowly. Write "Eat slowly, chew every bite 50 times" and put this reminder in many different places where it catches your eye – the table, the mirror, the refrigerator, the bathroom, etc.

Let us try to understand what obesity is. We associate it with an unsightly body shape, but first of all, it is an illness involving irregularities in many physiological processes taking place in the body. Like any other illness, obesity requires a long and tedious treatment. If obesity is neglected, it causes permanent damage to our health. Obesity affects all age groups, young and old. To fight an illness, we need to know its causes. In the case of obesity, the causes are our bad habits and addictions.

Stand naked in front of a mirror, take a close look at your body and notice all excess fat you carry around. Do not turn your head away; see what your gluttony and lack of strong will do to your body. What you see provides motivation to take some action.

Bad habits that lead people to obesity

Victor Hugo said that people couldn't achieve what they do not understand. To apply this rule to obesity, we cannot lose weight unless we understand what leads us to obesity.

Please pay close attention to the following list of bad habits that are largely responsible for leading people to obesity and try to eliminate these habits from your everyday life.

You will be pleasantly surprised by the results. Only your name will remind you of the obese person you once were.

1. **The habit of eating fast and not chewing the food well** causes poor digestion and the formation of fat layers in our body. Chew each bite at least fifty times – chewing is not a very demanding activity.

2. **Drinking fluids at meals** causes irregularities in the functioning of your digestive and hormonal systems. When you drink at meals, even water makes you fat. Drink at least twenty minutes before a meal or one to one and a half hours after a meal.

3. **Eating sweet baked goods** causes the absorbing walls of your digestive tract to be plugged up by starch and promotes the production of excess amounts of mucus in our body. Moreover, sweets promote weight gain. It is better to treat yourself to dried fruits, seeds (sunflower, pumpkin), and moderate amounts of nuts.

4. **The habit of frequent snacking or constant chewing** puts to much stress on certain systems in our body and takes them away from other important activities. As soon as anything gets into our mouth, the tongue (acting as the taste organ) sends a signal to our brain and

immediately many mechanisms are engaged. Among them, just in case, is our body's defense mechanism (the tongue does not provide full information about what it is that entered the mouth). Leukocytes have to leave their task of cleaning up and curing the body and they quickly gather around the stomach, where the content from the mouth is soon expected. When it is determined that no danger exists and leukocytes are not needed, they go back to their abandoned tasks. If there is another portion of food soon after, the whole process is repeated. As a result of being constantly overworked, leukocytes cannot do a good job at defending our body. This is why people who are used to frequent snacking are the first to get ill when there is, for example, a flu epidemic. Another problem created by constant snacking is the weakening of digestive enzymes produced by our body. Weaker enzymes mean incomplete digestion and the production of fat instead of water and carbon dioxide (by the way, chewing gum produces the same negative results).

5. Incorrect combining of food products makes digestion difficult and weakens the digestive mechanisms, because different foods need different digestive enzymes. Incorrect combining causes some food to putrefy and some to be turned into fat.

6. Lying down after meals activates mechanisms that normally function in sleep and takes the focus away from digestion. Undigested food is turned into fat. If possible do some walking on your heels after a meal to increase blood supply to the stomach and to improve digestion.

7. Sitting lifestyle does not use much energy and our body does not have the opportunity to use up its fat deposits. We should perform at least 1000 different energetic movements a day to increase the energy use.

8. The habit of eating while watching TV takes away the intimacy of our meals. Ancient dieticians advised that we should be "deaf and mute" at our meals. If we eat while watching TV, our brain gets confused – it has to process the information coming from the screen and to direct the digestive process at the same time. This interferes with our digestion and causes overeating.

9. Eating while irritated is another bad habit that causes us to forget moderation. Never eat under stress! Our liver reacts to stress first and the bile tubes become narrow. Bile does not get to our small intestine and food is not digested.

10. Eating before bedtime or at night is harmful because in sleep, all processes in our body are directed towards the rebuilding of cells and the rejuvenation of our entire body. The digestive organs do not have the necessary energy to process food at night. Eating at night gives us nothing but fat, liver stones, and kidney stones.

11. The habit of eating mostly refined and cooked food products makes us deficient in natural vitamins and microelements. We only get empty calories from these products; they do not have much nutritional value. Even if we eat large amounts, we still feel hungry and want to eat more. This way we end up eating five to ten times more than we should.

Now we can understand the cause of obesity. **When we lose the ability to properly process and absorb the food we eat, our body starts storing fat around our hips, thighs, belly, neck, etc. The psychological causes are more complicated. Most importantly, we have to understand that obesity is a disease and there is no excuse for tolerating it.**

How to lose weight?

When you remove the causes of your obesity, you will stop gaining weight. Then you still need to get rid of the excess weight you already have. It takes four steps:

1. Correct the alignment of lumbar vertebrae.
2. Gradually and systematically increase the amount of your physical activities.
3. Perform internal cleansing routines and go through regular fasts.
4. Combine food products correctly according to Table 2. (page 103)

1. Correcting the alignment of lumbar vertebrae

There are many methods of aligning the lumbar vertebrae. They are often easier to do than to describe; however, I am going to try anyway.

Exercise bar method. This is a simple and effective way to align the lumbar vertebrae. Grasp the bar with both hands (the bar should be adjusted for you so that your feet are about 4 inches (10cm) above the ground) and move your legs to stretch the lumbar spine. If you do not have an exercise bar, you can use the bough of a tree – simply hang from it on your hands to stretch the lumbar spine under your body weight.

String method. Put two chairs about 6 feet (1.8m) apart and join them with a string 2 feet (61cm) above the floor. Crouch on one side of the string, bend down your head, and move under the string to the other side and back; repeat two to three times.

Massage with the feet. Lie down on the floor belly-down. Get another person to sit down in a chair and gently massage your lumbar spine area with the feet. **Caution:** Never try to perform the massage by stepping on the lumbar spine area.

Massage with a roller. Wrap a roller in a soft towel and put it on the floor. Lie down with your lumbar spine area against the roller and slide your body back and forth (20-40 seconds in each direction). This method is painful but effective. At first, you will feel pain in the lumbar spine. After a few exercises (three to four days) the pain will start diminishing.

Manual therapy. There are many professionals lately that perform spine alignment procedures. The procedures are very effective as long as the person performing them is a good specialist. The best way to find one would be to rely on the opinion of other patients. **An improperly done procedure can leave you with an injury for the rest of your life.**

Now that you know what is to be done, start today and do not delay action until your vacation or other convenient time. **Your health cannot wait – it deserves your care every day.**

2. Gradually and systematically increase the amount of your physical activities

The human body is built in accordance with the physical and chemical laws. They are commonly known and scientifically proven. They are encoded in every nerve and muscle. They regulate the cells, tissues and bodily organs, assigning them specific functions.

If we recall our high school physics, we can understand how the above statement relates to the problem of obesity. The conservation of energy principle, one of the fundamental concepts of physics, declares:

> *Energy is neither created nor destroyed. It can only be converted from one form to another.*

Let us explain the connection. Energy contained in our food is used in life processes, e.g. for maintaining the body temperature or for digestion. Our hard working muscles can use up excess energy. If the muscles do not use this excess amount of energy, it is stored in fat for later use. We do not really need to use the somewhat foggy term "metabolism" when we talk about obesity. (As a biochemist, I still cannot fully explain what the term means.) Obesity can be treated as a disorder caused by the imbalance in the flow of energy. In physical terms, when the supply of energy is larger then its use (e.g. overeating accompanied by laziness and lack of exercise), fat tissue is formed to store the excess amount of energy.

Based on this reasoning, I have to repeat commonly known advice for obese people: Eat less and exercise more. As simple as it sounds, this is a sure and effective method of weight reduction.

3. Perform internal cleansing routines and go through regular fasts

The third step can be explained by a simple analogy taken from our everyday life. Everybody has used an electric pot for boiling water and has probably noticed that it takes less time and electric energy to boil water in a new pot. An older pot, whose heating element is covered with stone, needs more time and energy. To apply the analogy to our body, when it gets older and contains more unhealthy deposits (in the bones, muscles, circulatory system, lungs, etc.), it demands more food because of its inefficient use of energy. Increased consumption of food creates obesity.

This leads us to another conclusion: a sudden increase in weight is a signal of a large amount of unhealthy deposits inside our body. This should prompt us to go through the process of complete body cleansing. (See Complete Body Cleansing, page 175)

59

Regular short fasts are the best way to rejuvenate your metabolism. Your body will slowly get rid of its fat tissue and start digesting food the way it did in your younger years. Besides reducing your weight, there is another important benefit of fasting. When your body does not get any food, it starts looking for food in its own resources. First it consumes things that interfere with its functioning: ill cells, lumps, skin pockets, etc. In other words, it consumes its own diseases. It is not an accident that many religions prescribe fasting as a righteous act. It helps us to get rid of fat and at the same time purifies our mind and soul.

I want to stress I mean **fasting,** not food deprivation. There is a big psychological difference between food deprivation and fasting.

Food deprivation is a sudden and unexpected interruption in supply of nutrients to our body. It is as shocking for our body as a collision or a cataclysm.

When the body loses 20% of its weight because of food deprivation, it starts feeding on its own tissues. The process is destructive for both our physical and psychological health. Food deprivation is accompanied by fear and uncertainty. These two emotions turn off the immune system by blocking endorphins – hormones responsible for triggering the immune responses. The body becomes defenseless, weak, and unable to fight infections.

Fasting causes an entirely different reaction in our body. Fasting is a conscious, thought through, and well-planned temporary abstinence from food, preceded by a period of psychological preparation. There are two kinds of fasting:

Limited fasting – Eliminating intake of proteins and animal fat, e.g. drinking juices or eating fruits and vegetables only.

Strict fasting – Abstaining from all food and drink except water (including mineral water, in adequate amounts). It is most beneficial for improving your health.

When on total fasting, the body switches to endogenous (internal) food after 24-36 hours.

A person who is fasting is calm and able to focus on specific steps (described below); the body is able to make decisions based on a hierarchical system – it starts feeding on its own waste: disease-causing bacteria, salts accumulated in bones and joints, all kinds of cysts and lumps, cancerous cells, etc. In other words, it utilizes its own garbage. This is an amazing example of a natural healing power designed to cleanse the body of toxins in an effective and simple way. The main virtue of fasting (unlike food deprivation) is its power to cleanse our body and mind.

Some people start experiencing fatigue, nausea, or headaches after abstaining from food for eight to ten hours. Let us explain again why this happens and how it can be prevented.

As stated earlier, during fast the body feeds on its own toxins – this cannot be called good quality nutrition. Our blood absorbs toxic compounds from the large intestine and carries them throughout the body. Fatigue and headaches are results of autotoxication. How can we help our body remove the toxins quickly? We can help by performing an enema (important especially for those suffering from migraine headaches). **People who start their fasting with an enema never experience fatigue and hardly ever suffer from headaches.**

How to conduct a strict fast? Fasting can be short (1-3, 5, or 7 days) or long (9,11,14,17,21, or 40 days). Abstaining from food for more than 40 days turns the fast into food deprivation with all its harmful effects.

I will use my own schedule of fasting as an example:

• Every Tuesday and Friday,
• The first three days of each month,
• A seven-day fast every six months,
• Seven to eleven days of fasting once a year.

In total, I fast for 120 days out of the year. Such break from eating allows me to maintain a stable body weight and good overall health – I have no reason to complain.

If we fast for five or more days, the return to our usual diet should take as many days as the fast itself. We can drink freshly made juices and eat fresh or steamed vegetables on the first two days. Grains, plain yogurts or buttermilk can be added on the third day. The remaining items of our usual menu can be gradually re-introduced during days four and five.

61

How do I benefit from abstinence? I am not a slave of my own stomach – it does not direct my actions, as in the case of most people. We often see that people are ready to put everything aside (work, relaxation, love) in order to fill their stomach when it starts craving and making noises. This does not mean that I cannot enjoy a good tasty meal – to the contrary, I enjoy food very much. But I do not confuse enjoyment of tasty food with eating too much and too often. I follow the rule: **Eat to live instead of living to eat.**

I recommend the following schedule of fasting:

- 36 hours once a week,
- 48-72 hours once a month,
- 3-7 days once a year.

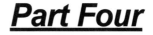

Part Four

"NATURAL DOCTORS" WHO ARE ALWAYS WITH YOU

In matters dealing with health, some of us are lazy (please take no offence) and some diligent. The lazy ones expect others to help them. They believe that taking care of their health is the responsibility of physicians. The diligent ones want to help themselves by discovering the real causes of their diseases but they do not always know how to do it. My books are intended mainly for the diligent people. The lazy ones should reflect on the old Eastern wisdom: "Nobody does anything for you without satisfying their own needs before yours." You ought not to thoughtlessly leave your most valuable things – your life and health – in somebody else's care. We spend our time in vain while we wait for a miraculous healing coming from somebody else – nobody can take better care of our health than ourselves. It takes strong will, persistency, diligence, knowledge, and experience to find our own way to good health. As we know, those who seek will always find.

Nature equipped all of us with defense mechanisms designed to protect our health. The stronger these defenses are the healthier our body is. Each of us has a different level of defensive abilities. They depend on our age, place and time of birth, the circumstances of our upbringing, our diet, etc. If our body has a low level of defensive abilities since birth, we can make a big difference just by adopting a lifestyle that follows the principles of nature.

There are twelve "natural doctors" that are close to us at any time of our everyday life, ready to help us without any charge, as long as we are willing and able to use their help. They are: our mind, light, air, water, food, physical exercise, heat, cold, sleep, rest, fasting, and urine. This book shows how to employ the help of some "healers." The information concerning the remaining ones is in the other books that follow. There are no superior and subordinate "healers." All of them are good, and we get best results when we comprehensively get help from them all.

PHYSICAL EXERCISE

Life is motion

Nothing causes as much damage to our body as long physical inactivity
— **Aristotle, an ancient Greek philosopher**

Physical effort is vital for the proper functioning of our heart, muscles, and circulatory system, for the effective removal of waste and toxins, and for the enhancement of our whole body's efficiency. Exercise helps us to better assimilate the energy we acquire from the natural environment. It is good for everybody – young and old. It is especially important for ill people. **An ill body needs much more physical activity than a healthy one.** Those who suffer from heart disease and circulatory problems or adversely react to barometric pressure changes, magnetic storms, solar radiation, etc. should regularly exercise and strengthen their body enough to withstand all these factors.

We should understand one simple truth: A physically active lifestyle not only protects us from becoming ill but also helps to eliminate many disorders we already have. What stops us from exercising? It is the old laziness.

If your way of thinking is "I have so many things to do, there is no time for exercise", it is time to change it. Convince yourself that exercise is as important as food for your muscles, internal organs, and brain. Physical inactivity makes us weak, ill, and prematurely aged.

Among the great variety of physical exercises, I would like to focus your attention on the healing walk, the healing run, and barefoot walk.

The healing walk

Walking is rightly called the king of exercise. No other exercise brings such harmony to the functioning of our muscles. It does not require any special attire or equipment; it can be done at any time and in any kind of weather. A daily walk, even 0.5 to 2 miles (0.8 to 3.2km) long, wonderfully stimulates our heart muscle and circulatory system. It is best to walk in the woods or a park; if that is not possible, we can even walk along a hall or balcony. During a walk, we should be relaxed and think about the fact that, with every step, our blood circulating through the blood vessels cleanses and nurtures our body. We can practice creating positive mental stereotypes by repeating, "I am healthy and strong, I am young and beautiful, I have a lot of energy" as we take each step. When we walk for healing, it is important not to become tired. We should feel light and refreshed. The intensity of the exercise can be increased slowly and gradually. For example:

Months 1-3:   A slow walk, 20-30 minutes twice a day
Months 4-6:   A fast walk 0.5-2 miles (0.8-3.2 km) every day
Months 7-12:   2.5-6 miles (4-10km) every day

The healing run

Spartans used to say: "If you want to be strong – run; if you want to be healthy – run; if you want to be wise – run."

The healing run strengthens the walls of our blood vessels, lowers blood pressure and cholesterol levels, enhances our gastrointestinal system, and strengthens the spine, joints, and muscles. Running is one of the best ways to build up our immunity against infections and to preserve our vigor and health. The benefits of running have been known for many years.

There have been examples of heart problems caused by intensive running exercises. However, the problems can only arise if we do not take into account our body's specific abilities and break the **rule of gradual increase in intensity, important in any physical exercises**. Some people's objective is not health improvement but quick weight loss. Their unfit and polluted body cannot bear the strain of intensive running exercise. **We should acquire the habit of moderation in everything – eating, drinking, exercising, etc.**

What rules should we follow in our running to feel refreshed, youthful, and healthy?

1. Use only well-fitting footwear with correctly shaped soles.
2. Run on the ground or grass – they absorb shocks; it strengthens your muscles and joints. Running on paved surfaces may cause damage and inflammation of your joints.

3. If you have not exercised much lately, run and walk alternately. Run 30 yards (27.5m) at a time and then walk for a while (do not strain your body).
4. Don't push yourself too much; relax your muscles and make your steps short. It is not distance that counts but the way all your muscles are exercised. The slight shocks on your heels move up the stream of blood in your veins. It works like a massage, strengthens the walls of your blood vessels, and prevents cholesterol and salts from forming deposits in your blood vessels and joints.
5. Dress warm in order to cause sweating – it helps in cleansing your body.
6. After exercising, lie down for about half the time you exercised. Place your legs above the heart level. In the standing position, 70% of the blood is below the heart level, and it is not easy for the heart to pump it upwards. When you run, your blood has to be pumped even faster. That is why you should let your heart rest after the exercise.
7. If you run in the evening, do it 2-3 hours after a meal.
8. Running should be a joyful exercise and not a chore.
9. It is better to exercise individually. Everybody's health and fitness are different and allow different speed and intensity of running. Beginners running with a group of well-exercised people, and trying to keep the same pace, can actually cause damage to their health.
10. Run every other day to maximize the healing effect of the exercise.

Walking barefoot

Unlike other mammals living on the Earth, humans walk on two legs. Our body acts like a battery with a positive charge in its upper parts including the head, and a negative charge in the lower body and legs. We get our positive charge from the universe and the negative one from the Earth. The higher the energy flow the healthier and more robust our body is. We acquire cosmic energy through breathing, contact with water (for example, when spending time at a lake or seashore), and eating plant-based foods. This is why we should maintain a close connection with air, water, and the world of plants. The charge from the Earth comes through our bare feet. Hippocrates wrote: "Best footwear is no footwear."

Studies have been done around the world on the processes stimulated in our body by walking barefoot. There are about 72,000 nerve endings on our feet – barefoot walking acts as a natural massage and positively influences the functioning of our internal organs. When we started using footwear, we reduced our connection with the electric charge of the Earth. This causes a wide range of disorders such as headaches, irritability, neurosis, coronary diseases, and many others.

During one of my trips to Tibet (high in the mountains), I noticed that children there go barefoot and lightly clothed, even in wet or cold weather. Amazingly, they do not catch colds or flu even when they are around people who are sick.

The way they looked was a testimony to their vibrant health – their muscles hard as steel, their skin silky-smooth, their cheeks rosy, their teeth strong and healthy.

Our ancestors did not have fancy footwear with soles made of synthetic materials. They spent most of their lives barefoot and this is why they enjoyed better health and stronger immunity than we do today.

We live in very different circumstances created by our advanced civilization and spending much time barefoot is impossible. Some of the things we can do is walking barefoot on the morning dew, sandy beach, or snow for 1-2 minutes every day, or putting our feet under a stream of cold water. That way we build up our immunity against colds, flu, and many other health conditions.

Going barefoot not only strengthens us and builds up our immunity but also prevents back, shoulder, and leg muscle pains suffered by those ladies who like wearing high-heeled and narrow-tipped footwear. This kind of footwear seriously retards blood circulation in the legs, causes stress and fatigue in the muscles (the foot support surface is reduced by 30-40%), and immobilizes the joints. The body posture caused by such footwear looks this way: the knees are slightly bent, the pelvis shifted back, and the torso shifted forward. The muscle group in the front is stretched and the one in the back is contracted. It is a violation against the spine and the entire muscular system of our body. I am not against elegance, but I would like to recommend (besides barefoot walks) a few prophylactic exercises that should help remove the resulting pain and feeling of heaviness in the legs and the entire

69

body. These exercises can also benefit those who spend a lot of time on their feet.

1. Take a piece of uneven and rough wood (carve it, if necessary) 2-3 inches (5-7.6cm) in diameter and, when you sit for a longer time (e.g. when watching TV), roll it under your feet.
2. Put hot and cold water in two basins. Hold your feet alternately in cold and hot water for about 30 seconds at a time (starting and ending in cold water), then dry and massage your feet and calf muscles. This procedure removes fatigue, stimulates blood vessels, and prevents varicose veins.
3. While you sit in a chair, raise your toes and rotate your feet in various directions with your heels on the floor.

Attention: Those who easily and frequently catch a cold should go barefoot or wear just their socks at home in the morning and in the evening 15-30 minutes each time. Increase the time by 10 minutes every day until it reaches one hour. After a month, they can go barefoot on the ground (back yard, park, etc.) When temperatures go down, they can go barefoot on frost for 30-60 seconds and then on snow for 1-2 minutes. Dry your feet thoroughly with a towel after each walk and put on a pair of warm socks.

No matter what your age is, take therapeutic barefoot walks as often as possible. You will notice positive changes to your health from day to day: increased energy, better sleep, cheerful spirit, and a renewed zest for life.

AIR

The breath of life

Our life involves constant processing of energy. The body needs energy to keep warm, process thoughts and feelings, fight diseases, build new cells, etc. – to do everything we collectively describe as life.

We know that we use about 50,000,000 kcal of energy from our birth to death. **The less energy we use in our life processes the longer we live.**

Most people believe that food is most important in providing us with energy. Nature, however, arranged it in a different way.

The simple fact is that we can survive several weeks without food, several days without water, but only a few minutes without air. That is why learning different breathing techniques is the best and the fastest way of maintaining good health.

Breathing exercises are vital because they allow us to absorb and retain huge resources of energy contained in the air. It is the reason why yoga masters put breathing techniques on top of their health ladder.

The objective of breathing exercises is to change our habitual way of breathing and to help our body retain carbon dioxide essential to the cellular metabolism (the exchange of gases between our cells and blood). Oxygen is used in oxidation reactions – this is why we should breathe clean, fresh air. Most of other chemical reactions taking place in our body depend on the concentration of carbon dioxide. If we take a very long walk (three to five hours) in the woods, and we breathe oxygen-rich air (especially when we breathe deeply), we may feel tired, heavy, and suffer from a headache. This happens because the concentration of carbon dioxide in our body becomes too low.

When we hold our breath for a while, the exchange of gases in our blood is better and there is more carbon dioxide necessary for cellular metabolism. This is another secret of good health and longevity.

Our breathing and aging

We can slow down our aging by breathing correctly. People who live long in different parts of the world explain their longevity by good physical condition and deep, cleansing breathing. Not many people are aware of this.

I once asked a Tibetan monk about the technique of deep, cleansing breathing. The only thing he said was: "If you want to live long, breathe deeply and infrequently."

It has been proven that we can extend our age by 10-20 years by a healthy diet; however, correct breathing can help extend it by 30-40 years. The Chinese, for example, suffer from fewer cancers than people in other parts of the world. Most of them are physically fit even at an old age. Daily breathing exercises play an important role in their good health condition. In contrast, many people instead of doing daily breathing exercises, breathe in poisonous cigarette smoke.

Breathing and smoking

The cells in a smokerís body suffer from constant oxygen deficiency and become oxygen-starved (hypoxic). The presence of hypoxic cells in our body creates an open gate for many diseases.

Two years of smoking ten cigarettes a day deposits 4.4lb (2kg) of toxic tar in a smokerís body. After ten years of smoking, the amount of tar grows to 8.8 lb (4kg). Those who smoke for over twenty years have over 13lb (6kg) of poisonous filth in their body. It is distributed in many places. Blood circulation disorders, digestive system problems, swollen veins in females, leg pains in males, and many other health problems are the consequences of taking pleasure in a few moments of smoking.

I often tried to help people quit the habit by the use of different methods: hypnosis, biotherapy, sometimes just a conversation. My experience tells me that it is best not to seek otherís help in quitting. We should try to help ourselves and remember that nobody else cares about our health as much as we do. If you are psychologically ready to quit smoking but lack the strong will to do it, I would like to offer you some helpful advice.

How to quit smoking? (For people who do not have a strong will)

1. Buy only one pack of cigarettes at a time.
2. Keep the pack out of your sight.
3. Smoke only filtered cigarettes.
4. Change the brand every two days.
5. Do not keep cigarettes on your desk at work.
6. Do not smoke when other people offer you cigarettes.
7. Do not carry a lighter or matches with you.
8. Clean your ashtray after every cigarette.
9. After the first puff, put your cigarette out for a while.
10. Do not smoke before breakfast.
11. Do not buy cartons of cigarettes.
12. Do not buy another pack until you finish the one you have.

13. Do not smoke for 15-20 minutes after meals.
14. Do not smoke inside your home.
15. Do not smoke during meals.
16. Do not smoke when you are out enjoying nature.
17. Do not smoke on holidays.
18. Do not smoke when others smoke.
19. Take three deep breaths before you light up.
20. Limit your smoking to less than one cigarette an hour.
21. Calculate how much money you spend on cigarettes in a week and a month.
22. Do a few exercises instead of having a cigarette.
23. Try to smoke without inhaling.
24. Write down reasons for quitting and read them daily before going to bed.
25. Reduce your smoking by one cigarette every day.

Correct breathing helps reduce your weight

Breathing and digestion are closely interconnected. Those of us, who are overweight, can get rid of the excess weight, without changing their diet, by breathing correctly.

We unnecessarily put strain on our body by the use of slimming diets or even worse – different artificial remedies and drugs. They can only bring temporary results. When we stop using them, the excess weight comes back. This kind of experimenting on our own body damages the liver, heart, and kidneys.

Those who would like to get rid of a few pounds can do it by holding their breath for 30 seconds several times a day. That way they can lose 4-9lb (1.8-4.1kg) in about two months. (And, of course, eating less is another important factor in weight reduction).

Breathing supplies oxygen to our body. The more oxygen our cells get, the less energy is wasted in the physiological processes. Oxygen brought in through our air passages only does not provide an adequate supply. This is why we should fully use another important breathing organ – our skin.

The total surface of our skin equals about 27 square feet (2.5 square meters). There is a constant gas exchange between our body and the environment through the pores of our skin.

This is why, whenever possible, we should let our skin come into contact with air, for example:

1. Spend time at home dressed (if possible) just in underwear.
2. Air your home several times a day.
3. Take walks before going to bed.
4. Spend more of your leisure time outdoors.
5. Spend as much time as possible at lakes or seashore.

Breathing for health

Ramacharaka, a great yoga master (from whom Europeans first learned the science of breathing) stressed, that regular breathing exercises completely eliminate the danger of respiratory system diseases, prevent us from colds and runny noses and improve the functioning of our digestive and nervous systems.

Even when an illness immobilizes us, we are still able to breathe and by breathing correctly, we can fight the disease.

Have you noticed that we breathe differently in different situations? For example, when we are nervous, our breath is shallow and more frequent. When we sing, we breathe in and then very slowly let air out. This brings the feeling of internal peace and relaxation. Laughter is very similar. We always laugh on exhaling. The diaphragm resists the exhaling action of the abdominal muscles to let the air out in small portions. This is why laughter is healthy for us.

Singing and laughter are the simplest yet the most effective breathing exercises and can become a significant part of our healthy lifestyle.

It seems that nobody needs to be taught how to breathe – we do it involuntarily by nature. However, lack of physical effort, spending most of our time indoors, obesity, and spine misalignments, caused our breathing patterns to change. In other words, we breathe the way we are able to, not the way we ought to. Only children up to the age of five breathe correctly, the way nature intended. Their way of breathing can be called full. We should practice full breathing before we start any other breathing exercises.

Full breathing

You can do the exercises in a standing, sitting, or lying down position. Your muscles should be relaxed and your eyes closed. Inhale slowly through your nose trying to fill the lower sections of your lungs first - the front of your abdomen should move forward. Then fill the middle sections of your lungs – the lower part of your rib cage should expand. Finally, the top sections of your lungs are filled, your rib cage moves upwards as the top ribs and the shoulders slightly expand.

Now try to join all three phases into one slow continuous inhaling that expands your rib cage from the bottom up and fills it with air. The air should be exhaled slowly through the nose while the chest is slightly inflated. As you exhale, your abdomen becomes gradually deflated.

If you find it difficult to learn the whole cycle by yourself, try watching a child breathe and copy what you have observed.

When you become familiar with the full breathing technique, you are ready to learn specific breathing rhythms.

By deliberately holding our breath, we can help to improve energy distribution in our body, enhance the functioning of the endocrine glands, regulate the heart rhythm, and increase oxygen level in our blood, which speeds up oxidation processes. It is no surprise that breathing exercises help us lose excess weight. If you spend 10 to 15 minutes of your time a day practicing full breathing, you may prolong your life by years.

Therapeutic breathing

It is best to do these exercises in the lying down position but if necessary, you can also sit down or stand up.

Inhale through your nose for 2 seconds, hold your breath for 8 seconds, and then let the air out through your nose for 4 seconds. The general pattern is 1:4:2 (inhale: hold: exhale). **Note:** The pause is 4 times longer and the exhaling 2 times longer than the inhaling. You can do this exercise for 2 minutes in the morning and in the evening.

Cleansing breathing

This kind of breathing cleanses the lungs, stimulates breathing centers, and helps to invigorate and regenerate our cells.

Breathe in for 2 seconds through your nose the same way you do in full breathing, hold your breath for 3 seconds, then move your lips forward and let a small stream of air out for 12 seconds. If there is still air in your lungs, let it out completely. Do this exercise in the morning and the evening - for 2 minutes each time.

Solar-Lunar breathing

Our daily breathing cycles depend on the influence of the Sun, the Moon, and the stars. Contemporary research shows that there are different rhythms of breathing involving the left and the right side of our nose and they change for a person during the 24-hour period.

It seems that our central nervous system regulates the air streams flowing through both nostrils and uses them for its own purposes. The air streams flowing through the right side influence the stimulating functions and the streams flowing through the left side influence the inhibiting functions.

For example, having your left nostril plugged and breathing only through the right side causes agitation and insomnia. Breathing only through the left nostril, with the right side plugged, brings constant fatigue.

Correct breathing through the nose is vital to our health. Yoga masters say: "To breathe through the mouth means to rush towards your death." I wholeheartedly agree with this statement.

When we breathe through our nose, 80% of dust and germs are stopped and neutralized by nasal mucous membrane. The nose acts as a gate that keeps all kinds of infections out of our air passages. When our nose is plugged and we breathe through the mouth, unfiltered air (with germs) gets into our larynx, trachea, and bronchi, causing inflammations not only in our air passages but also in the gastrointestinal tract. Children who breathe through the mouth have underdeveloped thyroid gland; their body develops slower; their digestive system malfunctions; they frequently get colds, flu or sore throat. Many kinds of bacterial infections (e.g. streptococcus, staphylococcus) are caused by unfiltered air getting in through the mouth.

Breathing through the mouth causes early aging, heart problems, and asthma in adults. We should learn to regulate our breath while we speak. Words should be spoken only while we exhale – that way we do not let air in through the mouth. For the same reason, we should not talk much at meals. It is best to eat slowly, be relaxed, and focus on chewing.

The technique that simulates solar and lunar influence on our breathing is as follows: Cover the right side of your nose with your right thumb, draw air in through the left side of your nose for 2 seconds, pause for 2 seconds and breathe out for 4 seconds. Then cover the left side of your nose the same way and perform the same exercise.

Repeat this exercise interchangeably 10-12 times for each side of your nose. This technique relaxes your nervous system, improves your mood, removes fatigue, and helps alleviate the symptoms of colds, rheumatic pains, and headaches.

The Vietnamese breathing technique

Breathe air in slowly through your nose and inflate your abdomen as much as possible, pause for 1-2 seconds, breathe out slowly and deflate your abdomen completely, then pause for 1-2 seconds. You can use the pattern: inhaling – 2 sec, pause – 2 sec, exhaling – 4 sec, pause – 2 sec.

You can do this exercise in series of 10 in the first week, 15 in the second week, and 20 in the third week. After a month, you can do 30-60 cycles depending on how you feel.

This technique is a wonderful massage of the intestines, liver, and pancreas.

Conclusion:
Breathing sustains our life. Correct breathing allows us to avoid diseases and maintain good health. We should perform breathing exercises twice a day – before breakfast in the morning and at least three hours after our last meal in the evening. It is best to exercise outdoors or in a well-aired room.

In all life situations, try to breathe through your nose as much as possible.

WATER

Water can be a remedy or a poison

Everybody wants to look young and live as long as possible. In order to achieve that, we follow different "miraculous" recipes and diets, buy expensive cosmetics, etc., but this is only a way to resist the symptoms of our aging. The real cause of the process is inside our body. One of the most important factors in our aging is the water we drink and use to prepare our meals.

The cells in our body (including blood) consist of 70% water; our brain is 90% water. The condition of our joints and blood vessels, the presence of liver and kidney stones, and the complexion of our skin depend on the quality of water we drink.

When we drink a lot of sweet beverages such as coffee, tea, pop, etc., we are treating our body as if it were a furnace where we can put anything and it will burn. We burn the years of our life when we do not respect the basic principles by which our body functions. If we do not appreciate the quality of fluids we drink, we shorten our life.

The water within our body

There are 130 kinds of water in nature. Water in our body's cells is under a special **structured** form. All other fluids that we consume must be purified and transformed into this specifically structured form. The process uses a significant amount of energy. For example, the processing of one liter of boiled water requires as much as 46 kcal. The energy necessary for processing all fluids we consume in our lifetime adds up to huge amounts. We must remember that our health depends on the amount of energy our body uses to service itself. The more energy is used for unnecessary water processing the less is left for repairing our cells and fighting diseases.

The water we drink

The water we drink contains large amounts of salts that are insoluble in our body. It is the same kind of salt that forms stones on the walls of our teapot. In addition, other harmful substances contained in water and the burned food pieces found in our soups get into our body and form harmful deposits that are hard to remove.

There may be traces of radioactive substances in tap water. Boiling does not remove them. We can get rid of other harmful substances by boiling our water, but at the same time we remove the active form of oxygen that is needed in our body. Boiling results in dead water because its structure is changed and it loses valuable biological information acquired from the Earth. This is why constant use of boiled water is not healthy for us.

Mineral water

Many people try using mineral water for both drinking and cooking. Mineral water contains certain salts and other substances that cannot be assimilated by our body. Some of these salts cannot even be removed. They can accumulate in our joints and cause their degeneration. After using mineral water for 2-4 weeks, we should quit doing so for 3-4 months. It is especially important for children – constant use of mineral water would cause them more harm than good. What kind of water is, then, good for us to drink?

Structured water

Structured water is most beneficial to our health. We can get it from fruits and vegetables, their juices, and from melted ice. Scientists became interested in the fact that the Yakut people of Siberia in northern Russia live, on the average, for one hundred years. They do not have running water or well water; they eat very little fruits and vegetables; their diet is poor in general but they virtually never get sick. The answer to the mystery turned out to be very simple. The Yakuts for centuries acquired their drinking water by cutting ice and letting it melt in the sunshine.

Water from ice

We know that aging begins with wrinkles. Wrinkling happens when our body's cells start to dry up. One of the main causes of aging is our body's inability to assimilate and process the water we consume.

The process of bone growth is finished when we become adults. The excess, unneeded amounts of calcium salts that we get from our food and water accumulate in our blood vessels and joints. This leads to irregular blood circulation, stones in our liver and kidneys, and gradual decline in the health of our entire body.

To slow down the aging process, we should learn to prepare and use water from melted ice.

Preparing structured water from melted ice

Structured water can be prepared from any kind of water. Pour water into a pot, cover the pot, put it in the freezer (25F/-4C) for 2 – 3 hours, then take it out and break the frozen surface. The water under the ice has the same structure as the water we have in our body's cells.

It is even simpler to prepare structured water in the wintertime. Put a pot with water outside. When it freezes completely, take it back in and let it melt slowly without warming it up. Drinking only one glass of such water every morning on an empty stomach can significantly improve your mood and the way you look. **It is especially beneficial for the elderly because it flushes not only unhealthy deposits out of their bodies but also old and dead cells, and this way it prevents them from cancers.**

How should we drink?

It is best to have half a glass or one glass of water when we wake up but first we should rinse out our mouth. We should use cold water melted from ice and swallow it in small gulps. Those who suffer from frequent constipation can drink cold structured water on an empty stomach to stimulate their large intestine.

Many people like to drink while they eat their meals. This is not advisable because water dilutes digestive juices in our stomach and that impedes digestion. **The habit of drinking at meals causes gas, bloating, constipation, and ulcerations of the digestive tract.** All fluids should be consumed 15-20 minutes before meals and at least one hour after meals.

To remove the feeling of dryness after a meal, rinse out your mouth a few times. If the dryness persists, eat an apple. It should be washed well and then eaten along with its peel, seeds and seed enclosures (everything that can be chewed up). The seeds and their enclosures contain much iodine and other elements essential for our body. It has been proven that six apple seeds contain our recommended daily intake of iodine.

How much water should we drink? The proper amount is different for everybody. The common opinion is that the average intake should be 60-75oz (2-2.5L) of all fluids. Others think that we should only drink when we feel thirsty and limit the amounts we drink at one time. There are many other schools of thought (sometimes contradictory) about the amount of water our body needs. For example, Yoga followers sip a little water every half an hour; the Tibetans drink only when they are thirsty; the French prefer wine to water. Every school of thought has its reasons. As a general guideline, I would like to quote an old Tibetan principle: Drink as much water as your body needs. If it gets too much, it knows how to get rid of the excess amount.

What is better: tea or coffee?

Both tea and coffee are beneficial as long as we use them in moderation: I would say one to two cups of tea or coffee a day. Such moderate amounts improve our blood circulation. They also energize our heart muscle, stimulate our brain, and relax our nervous system.

Green tea especially improves our health because it contains about 80 different elements necessary for our body. It strengthens our teeth, cleanses our blood, and unclogs the pores of our skin. It is a preventative remedy against stones in the liver, kidneys and bladder. It fights disease-causing bacteria. Do not make your green tea very strong – this may irritate your digestive tract. Other healthy beverages can be prepared by brewing the leaves of black current, raspberry, nettle, mint, balm, chamomile, etc.

The black varieties of tea are less beneficial because they contain substances that cause dryness in our digestive tract. To minimize the negative effects of these substances, we can add a bay leaf when we brew black tea. This will improve our tea's aroma and remove undesirable substances.

Freshly brewed tea has the best strengthening and invigorating effect. If we keep brewed tea for a few hours, it produces substances harmful to our health.

People have different tastes and habits. Some of us can do without any sugar; others must have sugar in their tea and coffee. At least half a teaspoon of unrefined sugar per cup should also be added to our tea to improve its quality. Raw sugar in small amounts is beneficial to our health.

A few remarks about sugar

White refined sugar is probably one of the most harmful products of our times. When used excessively, it ruins our general health by removing calcium and many other microelements from our body.

There is a recipe allowing us to change sugar-enemy into sugar-friend. Mix 27oz (750g) of white sugar with about 7 fl oz (200ml) of water (boiled or melted from ice) and 7 oz (200g) of honey in a glass jar. Keep it for eight days in room temperature, stirring it three times a day with a wooden spoon. The chemical reactions in the jar cause sucrose (responsible for absorbing calcium) to split into glucose and fructose – both very beneficial to our health.

Honey, raw sugar, or fruit products (jam, marmalade) are good substitutes for white sugar. From time to time, we should change the kind of sugar we use to sweeten our tea.

Water's memory

Water differs from other compounds found in nature by its ability to store information – water has memory.

As we already know, our cells consist of 70% water. Water in an ill organ contains information about the illness. Medication changes the structure of water for a while, but after the therapy, water still remembers the illness. This is just a simplified description – in reality the process is very complex and relies on thousands of different reactions. In order to understand the point, we do not need to analyze complicated formulas. Water's unique qualities have their advantages and disadvantages. The ability to perpetuate chronic illnesses by storing information about them is a disadvantage. How can we prevent it from happening? To remedy the problem, we can try to change the structure of water in our body. How to do it? None of the two methods mentioned below is a panacea; however some people who used them experienced a speedy health improvement.

1. For five months use only water acquired from melted ice for your drinking and cooking (fall and winter months).
2. Drink freshly prepared vegetable or fruit juices or juice blends, 2-4cups
   (0.5 -1L) a day (spring and summer months).

Juices can work miracles

Vegetable and fruit juices flush old and dead cells out of our body, help in dissolving salty build-ups, dissolve stones in our liver and kidneys, and play a role in preventing cancers. However, many people are concerned about chemicals used in the growing and storing of fruits and vegetables.

When we use a juicer, any chemicals that were used in the growing and storing of our fruits and vegetables get trapped in the pulp. The juice contains only structured water with dissolved vitamins, microelements, and easily absorbable mineral salts.

We should drink juices in small sips 20 minutes before a meal and hold each sip in the mouth for a few seconds. Enzymes present in our saliva digest carbohydrates contained in juices. If we drink fast (as most people do), the juices get directly to our stomach and undergo fermentation (our stomach's usual function is processing proteins).

A tip on preparing juices: We can put a filter (a double filter would be even better) on the opening of our juicer's tank to eliminate as many harmful chemicals as possible.

Freshly squeezed juices are the best

Chemical processing, preservatives, and pasteurization used in the production of juices not only destroy vitamins and microelements but also partially damage the structure of water along with the natural biological information recorded in it. The healthy ingredients last about four hours in fruit juices and ten hours in vegetable juices. Juices sold in stores, even if they are 100% natural, preserve only 60% of their nutritional value.

Synthetic vitamin C is often added to fruit and vegetable juices. The only thing it has in common with natural vitamin C is its chemical formula. There have been articles in scientific literature describing potential harmful effects of synthetic vitamin C. We should keep in mind that a glass of freshly squeezed juice contains many substances still unknown to science and prepared by the ultimate pharmacist – nature herself.

White sugar is added to most juices sold in stores. That is not a good idea. One of the main benefits of drinking freshly squeezed juices is the fact that they increase the alkalinity of our body, dissolve mucus and flush out insoluble harmful salts. In this way, fresh juices help cleanse our muscles, tissues, and blood. On the contrary, refined sugar increases the acidity of our body and causes fermentation in our intestines. This explains excessive gas and heartburn we often experience when we drink processed juices. Refined sugar added to juice is like "the spoon of tar that spoils the entire barrel of honey" in a Russian proverb.

The specific health benefits of each juice come from physiologically active substances produced by plants. Juices are so rich in microelements and minerals that they contain almost the entire periodic table of elements. In other words, all vitamins, microelements and minerals essential for our health are found in plant juices. One week of regular drinking of raw juices will bring a healthy complexion to your face, deep restful sleep, and better functioning of your gastrointestinal tract. The juices should be prepared from fresh healthy fruits or vegetables and consumed as soon as possible. When juices are stored (even if refrigerated), they undergo fermentation and decay, even though the taste may remain the same (beet juice is an exception).

Another good quality of plant-based juices is their easy assimilation by our body. Juices are assimilated completely 30 minutes after consumption, while even vegetable-based solid meals need one hour or more for digestion. Drinking juices provides relief for our digestive system and allows time for repairing and cleansing of all systems and organs with a minimal use of our body's energy.

There are three different ways to use "juice therapy"; depending on the objective, we have in mind:

1. Daily preventative use – up to 2 cups (0.5L)
2. Providing relief for our digestive system – 8-12 cups (2-3L) a day for 1-3 days (no longer)
3. As a remedy for a health problem – 2-4 cups (0.5-1L) a day for two weeks

Fruit & Vegetable juices – the source of health

Beet juice

Beet juice helps in the creation of red blood cells, improves blood structure, delays menopause in females, cures the diseases of circulatory system, digestive system, large intestine disorders, and dissolves stones in the liver, kidneys, and bladder (especially when used together with carrot juice). The proportion should be as follows: four units of carrot juice per one unit of beet juice. It can be used twice a day (one cup / 250ml at a time).
Note: We should not drink freshly squeezed beet juice (store in a dark place for 2-3 hours before consumption).

Carrot juice

Carrot juice contains vitamins A, B1, B2, B12, PP, K, E, and others. It improves the condition of our teeth, hair, and nails; removes the ulcerations of our stomach and duodenum; strengthens our immune system against present and future infections; positively affects our eyes and throat.

Many disorders of the liver and digestive system are caused by deficiency of certain elements that can be acquired from carrot juice. Various skin allergies, eczemas, rashes, and lymphatic system disorders disappear if you regularly drink fresh carrot juice.

Carrot juice promotes body cleansing; as a result many toxins overburden the liver.

A poorly functioning liver would not be able to handle on its own all the toxic substances that have to be removed from our body. They are transferred to the lymphatic system and then released through the pores in our skin.

The dissolved toxins are yellow or orange in color. If we have many toxic deposits in our body, our skin can turn yellow. It is a normal phenomenon and the skin will go back to its natural color once all toxic substances are discarded. In some cases, the process might take 6-12 months.

Carrot juice is similar to our blood in its structure and content, except that it has a magnesium atom in place of an iron atom. People in ancient times must have also noticed something extraordinary in carrot's "blood" – they often described carrot as king of vegetables.

One glass of carrot juice contains the entire recommended daily intake of all vitamins and microelements. They nurture our body and help regulate the functioning of our immune system. This way the immune system is able to fight even the most dangerous diseases. Some people are skeptical about the effectiveness of carrot juice therapy because it sounds too simple for them. Let's trust Einstein's opinion: **"Everything that is brilliant is simple."**

Fresh cabbage juice

Juice squeezed from fresh cabbage contains vitamin C and vitamins of B, K, and PP groups. It is a remedy for diabetes, gastritis, duodenum ulcerations, hemorrhoids, high blood pressure, obesity, and thyroid gland disorders. Compounds of sulfur, chlorine, and iodine contained in fresh cabbage juice cleanse our body.

One glass of cabbage juice in the morning and the evening allows us to lose excess weight because the juice causes intensive disintegration of fat tissue. However, if our intestines malfunction, cabbage juice may produce large amounts of gas. In such case, we should stop drinking cabbage juice until we clean our intestines.

Potato juice

Potato juice contains vitamins B and C, sulfur, phosphorus, potassium and other substances. It cleans bacteria out of our body, normalizes the functions of the digestive organs and the thyroid gland, removes various spots and rashes from our skin and face, and sometimes helps against strong headaches.

Some people suffer from stomach ulceration and they often try all kinds of remedies and therapies without result. I would like to suggest the following therapy: Drink about 3. 5 fl oz (100ml) of freshly squeezed raw potato juice in the morning on an empty stomach. Then lie down for half an hour with an electric pillow in order to warm up your stomach. The therapy should last 10-14 days. It cannot be interrupted for even one day.

Note: If you interrupt the therapy, start it over.

Cucumber juice

Cucumber juice is the best natural means to induce urination. It improves hair growth thanks to the high levels of silicon and sulfur. The juice contains elements necessary for life – 40% potassium, 10% sodium, 7.5% calcium, 20% phosphorus, and 7% chlorine. The high level of potassium makes it very valuable for people with high blood pressure. Our nails and hair particularly need the elements found in cucumber juice. You can drink half a glass a day of pure cucumber juice or, include it in a vegetable cocktail (see vegetable cocktails page 92).

Green pepper juice

Green pepper juice is rich in silicon, which is essential for our nails and hair. People suffering from excessive gas and frequent colic can get relief by drinking a glass of green pepper juice on an empty stomach in the morning.

Sorrel juice

Sorrel juice wonderfully regenerates the mucus layer in our intestines. It is rich in potassium oxalate, a compound very useful for our body in the organic form (when freshly prepared). It is better not to use sorrel in its cooked form very often because cooking changes the organic structure of potassium oxalate and then it may become a source of joint and muscle inflammations. Sorrel juice is also rich in iron and magnesium - elements needed in our blood. Phosphorus, sulfur, and silicon contained in sorrel juice are important for our entire body, head to toe. We can drink pure sorrel juice, but it is even better to add it to our salads.

Clover juice

Juice squeezed from cloverleaves is very helpful against female disorders, such as premature menopause. Scientists found clover to be a rich source of estrogen – female hormone made by the ovaries. Estrogen strengthens a female body, regulates the monthly period and prevents premature aging and decay processes.

Spinach juice

Spinach is very important for our digestive processes, starting in the stomach and ending in the large intestine. Raw spinach contains an organic substance that wonderfully cleans our intestines and improves their functioning. Two cups (half a liter) of properly prepared fresh spinach juice a day can help get rid of the worst forms of constipation within a few days or a few weeks.

The use of laxatives is often unwarranted. The way non-organic laxatives stimulate bowel movement irritates intestinal muscles. Because of their use, the system made up of local tissues, muscles and nerves remains idle, which causes the degeneration of our intestines.

Fresh juice squeezed from raw spinach is very effective in stimulating bowel movements and helps regenerate not only the intestines but also the entire digestive tract.

The consumption of refined sugar and other refined products, accompanied by vitamin C deficiency, cause gum bleeding and dental pulp diseases. The best remedy for these problems is a diet consisting of raw and natural plant-based foods, including adequate amounts of spinach and carrot juices.

If our body is deficient in elements found in raw carrot juice and spinach juice, we may suffer from a variety of health problems, such as ulcerations, anemia, nervous breakdown, irregular secretion from suprarenal glands and the thyroid gland, kidney inflammation, joint inflammation, furuncles, limb swelling, frequent hemorrhages, weakness, rheumatism, irregular heart function, low or high blood pressure, vision problems, and headaches (including migraine headaches).

Pumpkin juice

Pumpkin juice can help to induce urination in cases involving swelling of our body caused by heart and kidney disorders. It also strengthens the liver, stimulates the production of bile, calms the nervous system, and reduces fevers. The recommended amount is half a glass a day. Thanks to its high content of estrogen, pumpkin juice is very valuable in hormone-replacement therapy used by women going through menopause. Half a cup taken twice a day for a minimum of two months helps completely eliminate hot flushes, which put a lot of strain on a female body during menopause.

Watermelon juice

Watermelon juice not only has good thirst-quenching qualities, it also has medicinal qualities. It can be used as a urination-inducing remedy (in cases involving swelling), a preventative against arteriosclerosis, an aseptic (in case of heavy bleeding); it has an energizing effect (rich in sugars), rinses salts out of our body (kidney stones and gallstones), strengthens and cleanses our liver and kidneys. Drink about two glasses a day.

Tomato juice

Freshly squeezed tomato juice (unlike processed juice) contains certain types of phytochemicals that slow down fermentation and putrefaction processes in our intestines. High potassium content improves the heart function. The high content of malic acid stimulates metabolism. As far as vitamin C content is concerned, tomato juice is as rich as citrus fruits.

One glass of tomato juice covers half of our daily need for vitamins A and C. I recommend drinking one glass a day (pure juice or as part of vegetable cocktails).

Grape juice

Hippocrates, the father of medicine, greatly appreciated the health benefits of drinking grape juice. It refreshes and strengthens our body, fights bacteria, can be used to induce stools, perspiration and urination. The juice also lowers cholesterol levels and reduces blood pressure.

It is recommended to drink half a glass or a glass of grape juice daily, one hour before a meal.

If we regularly drink grape juice, it is better not to drink any milk or eat any fresh fruits because it would cause fermentation in our intestines. Those who suffer from diabetes, obesity, or ulcerations of the stomach and duodenum should not drink grape juice in large amounts.

Lemon juice

Lemon juice is rich in vitamin C, microelements and hormones. It wonderfully cleans insoluble salts and slime out of our body. **Drinking juice squeezed from one lemon every day helps us stay young.** It contains estrogen-like phytochemical substances and therefore is very beneficial for older females. Some chemical compounds found in lemon juice are very effective in the prevention of infectious diseases. **We should drink lemon juice as a preventative measure against the flu epidemic and colds in late fall and early spring.**

Lemon juice can be used in a preventative or a healing therapy. For prevention, it is used in the following dosages:

Day 1 – 1 lemon – Day 10
Day 2 – 2 lemons – Day 9
Day 3 – 3 lemons – Day 8
Day 4 – 4 lemons – Day 7
Day 5 – 5 lemons – Day 6

From the first to the fifth day, we add one lemon every day and from the sixth to the tenth day, we subtract one lemon a day. In total, we drink juice squeezed from 30 lemons during ten days.

We can prepare lemon juice in the following way: Cut a lemon in half horizontally, squeeze both halves and drink the juice without adding any sugar. If you are not able to drink pure lemon juice, dilute it with water and add one teaspoon of honey. You should not discard the squeezed lemon – it contains valuable phytochemical ingredients and essential oils that are beneficial for the heart, blood vessels and brain. Cut the squeezed lemon into small pieces, put them in a jar, add honey or sugar, and put in the refrigerator. In ten hours, you will have an excellent lemon extract that can be mixed with boiled or mineral water and used instead of tea or coffee.

For a description of lemon juice healing therapy, look in "Osteoporosis – Questions and Answers" (page 161).

Garlic juice

Garlic juice was used as a remedy in ancient Greece. It induces appetite, improves digestion, helps against respiratory system diseases, prevents colds, fights headaches and insomnia, induces urination, clears the throat, and reduces pain. In the case of chronic insomnia, it is enough to drink 3. 5 fl oz (100ml) of boiled water mixed with one teaspoon of honey and juice squeezed from one garlic clove for a few days, to return to regular sleep pattern. To stop a strong toothache, we can put pulp made from a garlic clove on the left wrist and wrap it with a bandaid (for 3 to 5 min.) There are at least two natural antibiotics in garlic effective against about thirty kinds of disease-causing bacteria. Phytochemicals found in garlic are able to completely stop fermentation and putrefaction processes in our intestines. Garlic contains germanium that effectively fights heart diseases and blood vessel disorders. We can completely cure dysbacteriosis (the degeneration of large intestine's microflora), a disorder affecting about 90% of children and adults, by taking garlic juice for just two weeks.

A recipe for "the elixir of youth", a type of garlic extract, was found in 1971 by a UNESCO team in a Tibetan monastery and was dated about 4-5 centuries B.C. The extract cleans accumulated fat out of the body, rinses out insoluble calcium, radically improves metabolism, cleanses blood vessels, prevents heart attacks, arteriosclerosis, and paralysis, removes the sensation of buzzing from the head, improves sight, and regenerates the entire body.

Garlic extract. Take 12oz (350g) of peeled, freshly harvested garlic, crush it into a pulp, and mix with 7 fl oz (200ml) of vodka (40% proof and up). Close tightly in a jar and put in a dark, cool place (do not refrigerate) for 10 days. Then strain the pulp, put the fluid in a jar and keep it in a dark place for another 4 days. Now it is ready.

Use the extract according to the following dosage:

Day	Breakfast	Lunch	Dinner
1	1 drop	2 drops	3 drops
2	4 drops	5 drops	6 drops
3	7 drops	8 drops	9 drops
4	10 drops	11 drops	12 drops
5	13 drops	14 drops	15 drops
6	16 drops	17 drops	18 drops
7	19 drops	20 drops	21 drops
8	22 drops	23 drops	24 drops

9	25 drops	25 drops	25 drops
10	25 drops	25 drops	25 drops
11	25 drops	25 drops	25 drops

After this, take 25 drops three times a day until all extract is used up. Each amount of the extract should be taken with 1.7 fl oz (50ml) of plain yogurt or kefir.

Many people dislike the intensive smell of garlic. To get rid of the smell, chew on a parsley, an apple, a lemon peel, or an orange peel.

Caution – Use the garlic extract therapy only once a year.

Cocktails that heal

I suggest a few kinds of vegetable cocktails that have helped many people deal with persistent health problems. As we know, many diseases are linked to deficiency in minerals. Vegetable cocktails replenish the levels of minerals in our body.

Calculate the amounts of ingredients based on the following proportions to produce the desired amount of vegetable juice blend.

Cocktail number 1

Blend carrot juice, cucumber juice and green pepper juice in proportion 4:1:1 (e.g. 4 cups + 1 cup + 1 cup or 1000ml+250ml+250ml).
Usage: rheumatism, bone and muscle pain, limb swelling

Cocktail number 2

Blend carrot juice, cucumber juice and lettuce juice in proportion 4:1:1 (e.g. 4 cups + 1 cup + 1 cup or 1000ml+250ml+250ml).
Usage: skin diseases, eczemas, rashes, pimples, eye inflammations, and tender nails

Cocktail number 3

Blend carrot juice and spinach juice in proportion 1:2 (e.g. 1 cup + 2 cups or 250ml + 500ml).
Usage: abdominal pains, cramps, excessive gas, constipation, rheumatism, anemia, low or high blood pressure, migraine headaches

Cocktail number 4

Blend of carrot juice and green pepper juice in proportion 1:2 (e.g. 1 cup + 2 cups or 250ml + 500ml).
Usage: skin spots and discoloring often affecting the elderly

Cocktail number 5

Blend carrot juice and parsnips 2:1 (e.g. 2 cups + 1 cup or 500ml + 250ml).
Usage: genital-urinary system inflammations, eye inflammations, and inefficient blood vessels

Cocktail number 6

Blend tomato juice, apple juice, pumpkin juice, and lemon juice in proportion 2:4:2:1 (e.g. 2 cups +4 cups +2 cups +1 cup or 500ml + 1000ml + 500ml + 250ml).
Usage: cleansing mucus out of the body, disintegrating fat tissue; it brings wonderful results when used for digestive system relief (1.5-2 L a day).

Cocktail number 7

Blend cucumber juice, blackcurrant juice, apple juice, and grapefruit juice in proportion 2:2:1:1 (e.g. 2 cups +2 cups +1 cup +1 cup or 500ml + 500ml + 250ml +250ml).
Usage: for fresh and attractive skin, a calm and strong nervous system, good brain and memory function, stronger immune system. One cup provides the recommended daily intake of vitamin C.

Juice therapy dissolving calcium stones

Stones and sand in our gallbladder and kidneys are the result of our body's inability to remove deposits of non-organic calcium. This form of calcium comes from the consumption of refined and processed foods.

Calcium, the element essential for our body, comes in two forms – organic and non-organic. Organic calcium is the form that dissolves in water. Blood carries calcium to our liver, where it is completely assimilated. Organic calcium is found only in raw fruits and vegetables, their juices, and those dairy products that do not undergo thermo-processing (homemade cheese, plain yogurt etc.)

Calcium contained in processed foods (bread, buns, pastries, sweets, chips, fries, flour-based products etc.) is in non-organic form, does not dissolve in water, and is treated as a foreign substance by our body. Insoluble calcium forms gallstones, causes hemorrhoids in the rectum, stones and sand in the kidneys, and cancer in the stomach.

The main cause of stones in our gallbladder and kidneys is our excessive consumption of baked goods, sweets, pasta, over-cooked grains, and other refined flour-based products.

Centuries of experience in natural therapy teach that surgical removal of stones (in most cases) does not make sense. The rational use of natural therapies brings much more desirable results. People who suffer from stones in their gallbladder and kidneys must understand that surgery removes only the effect while it is necessary to deal with the cause of the problem. We already know what the cause is.

To get rid of stones in your gallbladder and kidneys, use the following therapy (in detail):

Drink juice squeezed from one lemon blended with half a glass of hot water 3-4 times a day. In addition, have a blend of equal amounts of carrot juice, beet juice and cucumber juice 3-4 times a day, half a glass each time. The therapy can last a few days or a few weeks, depending on the amount and the size of stones. During the therapy, eliminate flour-based products, sugar, grains, and dairy products (except butter) from your diet.

HEAT AND COLD

The healing water

Each organism begins its life in water; a human fetus is no exception. Kneip, a German physician, wrote: "Each contact with water means an additional minute in our life." Recent scientific research proves that our body can most easily rebuilt its natural electric potential with the help of water. It is no coincidence that many cultures' customs include rituals such as offering water to travelers or baptizing babies with water. Both Hippocrates in ancient Greece and Avicenna, an Arabian physician and philosopher in medieval times, extensively used water therapy by applying alternately cold and hot water and then massaging a patient's body. This kind of therapy improves blood circulation and metabolism, helps to flush mucus out of the body, and consequently causes a speedy healing process. People are often ready to travel hundreds of miles looking for a miraculous cure but they do not realize that better results can be achieved using regular water flowing out of their tap.

Seneca, a great philosopher, was right when he remarked that the essence of things is very simple. It turns out that by simply applying cold and hot water we can get unexpectedly good results in fighting many diseases. The importance of the alternate use of cold and heat lies in the fact that heat stimulates the surface areas of our body and increases blood supply to the skin while cold stimulates blood circulation in our internal organs. By doing so, the alternate action of cold and heat in water therapy becomes a miraculous cure for many diseases because it regulates blood circulation, strengthens our muscles and heart, and improves our immune system.

Alternate cold and warm massage decreases our body's sensitivity to cold and heat and refreshes our nervous system. It is particularly advisable for elderly people because it decreases their proneness to fatigue and sweating, the sensitivity of their muscles and joints, and their reaction to weather changes. The effects are even better if extracts of chamomile, sage, or other medicinal herbs are added to water used in the massage. This provides a double benefit for wilted skin – the benefits of the massage and of the vitamins contained in the extracts. Soak a small towel in cold water, wring it out and massage one of your arms. The same routine should be repeated for the other arm, the chest, back, and legs. The total time for the entire body should be 3-5 minutes. Then massage with a dry towel until the skin feels warm and turns red. It is best to use this therapy every morning after an alternate cold and hot shower.

Alternate hot and cold shower is recommended in the morning and the evening every day. Adjust the water temperature to make it comfortable and pleasant for 40 seconds. Use the cold-water knob to decrease the temperature (within the comfort zone) for 20 seconds, and then increase it again using the same knob. Follow the pattern: 40 seconds – warm, 20 seconds – cold. Repeat for 3-8 minutes, depending on how you feel.

Note: When you shower in hot water, start from your head; when you turn on cold water, shower your legs first and then the upper body. Always end with a cold shower to let your blood vessels contract and to prevent colds. During cold seasons, do not go outdoors for about 40 minutes after your alternate hot-cold showers.

Therapeutic baths at home

Therapeutic baths are one of the oldest methods of healing. They are easy to prepare and yet they bring us many benefits, such as removing fatigue, calming our nervous system, regenerating our skin, improving our sleep, increasing metabolism, and removing pain and stress from our muscles. You can enrich your bath water with herb extracts for unique scent. Many people with back or arm pain think of visiting a healer or traveling to some mineral springs for therapy. These plans often remain unrealized for various reasons, including financial difficulties, and we keep suffering from our pains. In this situation, using our regular bathtub at home can prove just as effective. We have to keep in mind that, to be effective, home therapeutic baths must be done in a series - one bath done every other day for two or three weeks. We don't need anything special to prepare a bath. In order to relax better we can listen to our favorite music. A therapeutic bath brings the feeling of relaxation and enjoyment because by cleansing our body it also clears our mind. A bath can last 15-25 minutes, depending on how we feel.

Bath number 1 (temp. 93-98.6F/35C-37C)

Pour 5 quarts (5L) of boiling water on 0.66lb (300g) of chamomile flowers, set aside for 2 hours, strain, and then pour into your bath water.
Usage: For the relief of back pain, joint pain, and inflammations; for general rejuvenation

Bath number 2 (temp. 93F/34C)

Pour 5 quarts (5L) of boiling water on 0.44lb(200g) of sage flowers, set aside for 2 hours, strain, and then pour into your bath water.
Usage: To relieve low blood pressure, asthma, bronchitis, skin disorders, inflammations, and joint problems

Bath number 3 (temp. 100F/38C)

Put 3.3lb (1.5kg) of spruce branches in 5 quarts (about 5L) of water and boil for 30 minutes; strain and pour into your bath water.
Usage: To relieve back and bone pain, limb swelling

Bath number 4 (temp. 98-100F/37C-38C)

Put 4.4lb (2kg) of regular, iodized salt in your bath water. Make sure it is completely dissolved.
Usage: To calm the nervous system, cleanse and rejuvenate the skin, remove muscle and joint pain, and improve the immune system

The description of water therapies would not be complete without mentioning the sauna, a wonderful invention of our ancestors that can help us improve both our physical and psychological wellbeing.

The wonderful power of sauna

When we ask people, what is most important for them, they usually mention two things: good health and long life. Good health is a gift of nature but it is up to us to claim it. We can achieve good health in many ways as long as we are not hesitant to make the first step.

Take a look at people walking in the streets – their joints move with difficulty, their feet hardly lift off the ground, their knees do not bend much, and their spine and neck seem as stiff as a wooden stick. Almost everybody we know complains about back pain. The majority of people experience pain in their shoulders and arms when they get up in the morning. It is usually blamed on one factor: our joints hurt because we are aging. This is not the case. Nature provided our joints with the means to be flexible in the form of a special substance, a kind of lubricant. The amount of that lubricant does not decrease by itself, no matter the age. The loss of flexibility in our joints really results from the presence of various toxic salts in our skeletal system. Sauna is one of the most effective and pleasant methods of cleansing accumulated toxins out of our skin and internal organs.

Build up your immunity!

Scientific data show that people who use saunas get flu and colds ten times less than the average. We know that weather influences our health. Our body is influenced by temperature and humidity changes, winds, magnetic storms, etc. If our body's defensive mechanisms are weak, we immediately feel adverse effects of weather changes on our health. Sauna is an excellent way to make our immune system stronger by the use of cool, hot, humid, and dry stimulants. Our body experiences constant changes of surrounding temperature: 68-75F (20-24C) when we undress, 176-212F (80-100C) when we enter sauna, 86-104F (30-40C) in a hot shower, and 59-68F (15-20C) in a cool shower. Such alternately hot and cold shower is the best thermo-massage for the blood vessels of our skin and muscles. A hot shower expands blood vessels, while a cold shower produces the opposite (contracting) effect. This kind of therapy makes us immune to any weather changes.

Who can use sauna?

We know that prevention and immunity building are good concepts. We all agree with that, but we often find convenient excuses not to use these simple concepts in our life. The use of sauna does not require any effort and is beneficial for everybody – young or old, for those in good health as well as for those who are ill (with some exceptions mentioned in the next paragraph). There is a saying in Finland: "Everybody who can walk to the sauna can use it."

Sauna and your heart

Swiss doctors use saunas in the treatment of high blood pressure. In most cases, it takes only 15 sessions in sauna to bring blood pressure back to normal. They proved that sauna helps regulate our blood pressure – decreases, increases, or stabilizes it according to need. People with heart defects should remember that our blood circulation is affected by not only temperature changes but also by humidity and the length of time spent in sauna. **Please consult your physician before you decide to try the power of sauna.**

The calming sauna

It is believed that one out of four people suffers from some form of insomnia. Our biological clock ticks irregularly as a result of an unhealthy lifestyle – night eating, stress, coffee consumption, smoking, medication overuse, etc. French scientists noticed that sauna is also an excellent remedy for insomnia.

The Finnish, who use saunas daily, say: "Anger and hatred burn out in sauna." This effect is produced by the state of calmness, relaxation, and pleasure that we experience. The warming of our muscles and bodily organs relieves pain in our bones and joints. It improves our mood and helps us forget our troubling thoughts and daily worries – temperature changes are a good means of decreasing nervous tension. I recommend sauna for everybody, even if you do not come from a culture where using saunas is a common practice. If you use sauna regularly, it will become a habit – it is a simple and well-tested method to maintain good health.

Cleansing effects of sauna

Most food products in today's world contain large amounts of preservatives, food coloring, and salt. It is unfortunate that such substances get into our body along with food. Intensive sweating in the sauna allows our body to get rid of these substances. It relieves our kidneys because through sweating we can discard three quarters of all toxins accumulated in our body. One hour of heavy sweating in sauna can discard as much toxic material as a set of healthy kidneys in 24 hours. Improved metabolism helps us lose excess weight.

The power of sauna

German researchers noticed that women who use sauna regularly during their pregnancy have an uncomplicated and speedy delivery. The babies' health was monitored for the next three years, and they showed very good immunity to infections and colds. In addition, nursing mothers who use sauna produce more milk.

It is customary for children in Finland, Germany, and Russia to use saunas along with their parents as a cure and a method to build up immunity. Sauna prevents them from illnesses caused by changes in temperature and humidity. In Germany and the Czech Republic sauna use is included in school and daycare programs.

Note: Children between the ages of three and twelve can stay in sauna 1.5-3 minutes at a time in the temperatures of 122-140F (50-60C) and humidity of 25%.

Sauna and your skin

Skin protects our body from harmful factors in our environment. A significant part of our breathing is done through the pores in our skin, and nothing clears the pores as well as using sauna.

Our skin acts as a double filter: it discards harmful toxins from the body and absorbs healthy substances into it. We can make use of this quality by including aromatic oils in our therapy. The oils are absorbed both through our air passages and the widened pores in our skin. They positively influence the function of our nervous system, heart, liver, and blood vessels (eucalyptus helps against sore throat and runny nose; chamomile helps against insomnia; mint alleviates digestive tract pains; lavender and jasmine stimulate our brain; pine oil is very helpful in calming our nervous system).

If we suffer from pimples, acne, rashes, etc., we can use a solution of one tablespoon of salt and one tablespoon of baking soda in a glass of water to cure the problem. Rub the solution on your skin (except for the face) before you enter sauna, and rinse it off with warm water when you leave sauna.

What should we drink in the sauna?

Some experts recommend cold drinks in sauna for quenching thirst, while others recommend hot tea. American scientists conducted a study in which one group of participants drank cold beverages and the other drank hot tea. The study proved that cold beverages lower the temperature just in the mouth, while hot tea lowers the temperature of the entire body by about 1.8-3.6 degrees Fahrenheit (1-2 degrees Celsius). It works even better when we add a few leaves of blackcurrant, raspberry, wild blueberry, and a little bit of honey to our tea. The tea should be freshly brewed (brewing time: 4-6 minutes). If it is not fresh, it no longer contains many useful substances.

Important details:

1. The optimal time to stay in sauna is 5-10 minutes.
2. Rest for 10-15 minutes after each stay in sauna.
3. The number of stays in sauna should be limited to:
   - 2-3 for adults
   - 1 for children age 3-12 (can stay in the sauna 1.5-3 minutes at a time)
4. The most beneficial temperatures:
   - 50-60C (122-140F) and humidity of 25% for children
   - 60-70C (140-158F) for those over 50 years of age
   - 90-100C (194-212F) for everybody else
5. Hot tea and juices are the best drinks in sauna and during breaks.
6. It is a good idea to massage your feet and hands in sauna.
7. You can put your feet in a basin with warm water while in sauna to increase the weight reduction effect.
8. Do not put any lotion on your skin or body while in sauna.
9. Take a warm and then a cold shower each time you exit sauna; do not towel dry your skin.
10. Do not eat much when you are about to use sauna; do not drink any coffee or alcohol.

FOOD

Together or separately?

Let's take a close look at ourselves – it is hard to find a completely healthy person after the magic age of forty. In a typical family, the grandma suffers from constant pains in her bones and joints; her eyesight is poor. The grandpa has heart problems, digestive system disorders, or asthma. The father complaints about indigestion and back pains; mom suffers frequent constipation and headaches. Children wear glasses, suffer from allergies, have acne, and often get colds or runny noses.

Television commercials advertise "miraculous" remedies for acne, tooth decay, joint pain, colds, etc. **In reality, all of these remedies only fight visible symptoms whose real causes remain within our body.** It is a shame many adults do not understand this truth and, to express their affection, treat children to ice cream, sweet beverages, candy, and other products full of sugar. All these products turn into poisons in them for the rest of their lives. **When I hear discussions about hereditary diseases, I often want to say that diseases are not inherited. We inherit an unhealthy lifestyle.**

Plants and animals living on our planet offer us a huge variety of foods. The fundamental question is how to choose products that are really essential for our body. One of our most common and serious misconceptions is the idea that combining many different products in our meals helps us maintain good health. It is also a common belief that meals rich in animal proteins are nutritious. Ironically, this kind of food is often the source of our discomfort and illness.

For example, our meal often consists of a soup, steak, fries, and a sweet beverage, fruit or some other dessert. As we know, all of these products require different digestion times and different digestive juices. They create a mixture that is hard to digest and our stomach does not know where to start. Fruits start decomposing in the stomach and produce poisons such as alcohols and acetic acid. The combination of meat and potatoes produces solanine - a highly toxic substance. It all happens in our stomach, where it is humid and warm. (Remember how wine is made at home – cut-up fruits and some sugar are placed in a jug and kept in a dark place where they start to ferment.) It is no surprise that such meal causes gas, stomach pain, and the feeling of heaviness in our entire body.

Improperly combined meals cause putrefaction processes in our body. They produce hydrogen sulfide and phenol – both of them strong poisons. All poisons should be discarded with our urine. However, if we load meat in our stomach every day, our body cannot keep up with the need to neutralize poisons.

We often behave as if our stomach was a bag able to accept everything thrown into it (some nutrition theories want us to believe that). In reality, that bag becomes ill and weak. Our body starts resembling a time bomb that is going to explode by the time we are fifty and may cause the following health problems: heart disease, high blood pressure, arteriosclerosis, diabetes, blood clots, asthma, allergies, digestive system disorders, hormonal disorders (females), and impotency (males). To avoid all these health problems, we should carefully analyze mistakes we make in preparing our meals.

Hippocrates maintained that food should be our medicine. In order to implement this piece of wisdom in our life, we have to change our eating habits and start observing certain principles. These principles are the topic of the following segment.

Properly combined foods

Food products can be divided into the following groups: proteins, carbohydrates, fats, fruits and vegetables. The principles of combining these food groups are described below.

Table 2. Combining food products.

PROTEIN RICH FOODS	FATS AND "LIVE" PRODUCTS	CARBOHYDRATE FOODS
Meat and meat soups, fish, eggs, eggplant, beans, Windsor beans, nuts, sunflower seeds, plain yogurt, kefir, cottage cheese, buttermilk	Grease, butter, vegetable oil, fruits (raw or dried), vegetables (raw or dried, except potatoes), fruit and vegetable juices. It is better to always consume milk, dry wine, melon and banana separately from other products	Breads and other flour based products, grains, potatoes, sugar, honey, products containing sugar, pasta, jams, candies

   └ Can be combined ┘ └ Can be combined ┘

Foods in the middle column can be combined with either protein foods in the first or carbohydrate foods in the third column, but foods in the first and the third columns should never be combined.

These rules for combining foods may be hard to accept for some people, because they are used to eating meat with bread, buns, potatoes, or rice.

103

If you try observing the rules for just one week, you will notice that you eat less and have a lot of energy. You will require less sleep to feel well rested. Your mood will be balanced, and you will feel calmer. The rules for combining food products are not complicated. It is a good idea to pay attention to them.

The principles of eating protein rich foods

1. If you combine proteins with fats (e.g. meat fried in vegetable oil), always eat plenty of vegetables. Large amounts of vegetables prevent fats from impeding the digestion of proteins.
2. It is better to eat only one kind of protein food at a meal - e.g. only meat or only fish or only peas.
3. Proteins should preferably be eaten for supper, at least two hours before bedtime. Our body repairs its cells at night and uses proteins in the process. A vegetable salad should precede every protein meal.

Examples:

- Vegetable salad and cooked meat or burgers
- Vegetable salad and cottage cheese
- Vegetable salad and cooked beans or peas

Some useful advice:

- It is best to prepare meat in the oven or on a grill rather than cook or fry it on a pan.
- Meat soups need thirty times as much energy for digestion as meat. As I mentioned before, meat products contain over twenty different toxic substances. When we cook meat, these substances can be found in our meat soup. This way our soup is full of toxins coming from a dead animal. It is a good idea to completely eliminate meat soups from our diet.
- We do not need proteins in large amounts. It is enough to eat meat, fish, or poultry just twice a week. Animal proteins can be fully substituted – 3.5oz (100g) of nuts meets our daily protein requirement; 4oz (120g) of beans or peas can replace 7oz (200g) of meat or 10.6oz (300g) of fish.

- Meat and fish should only be eaten fresh – do not put them away for the next day.
- When you cook meat, put a piece of apple in the pot ten minutes before you take the meat out - this will make your meat juicier. To make your cooked fish tastier, add cold water to the pot a few times while you cook.

The principles of eating carbohydrates

1. Eat one kind of starch at a time. Combining different type of starch increases our appetite and leads to overeating.
2. Combining flour-based products and grains with jam or sugar causes fermentation in the stomach. This is why we experience heartburn after eating sweet buns and jam-filled baked goods. Do not combine starchy foods with sugars (e.g. grains with sugar). Honey can be eaten with bread but it is better to drink it dissolved in warm boiled water.
3. Dried sweet fruits can be combined with starchy foods: bread, grains or rice.
4. Grains, bread, potatoes, and other starchy foods should not be combined with protein foods such as meat, fish, eggs, or cheese. The interval between consuming carbohydrates and proteins should be at least 2-3 hours.
5. The best time to eat starchy foods is between 9 a.m. and 1 p.m. because we get most of our energy from carbohydrates. This energy is used up in our daily activities. Those who gain weight easily should especially pay attention to this rule in order to avoid obesity.
6. A vegetable salad should be eaten before starchy foods.
7. The best kind of salad is one consisting of cabbage, carrot, raw or cooked beets, dill, parsley, some salt and other seasoning. Enzymes found in vegetables help in digesting starch.

Some useful advice:

- The digestion of starch begins in the mouth – starchy foods should be chewed thoroughly.

- Grains and yeast-free baked goods are rich in fiber – they clean our digestive tract. If we want to maintain our digestive tract in perfect order, we should eat them every day.
- The healthiest types of grains are buckwheat, wheat, corn, barley, and rice (especially wild, unrefined). It is better to cook grains with small amounts of water. One third of our diet should consist of grains.
- When cooking grains it is best to use the interrupted cooking method.

  For example, buckwheat can be prepared in the following way:
  - Rinse the buckwheat and soak it for 3-4 hours
  - Do not change the water; cook buckwheat for 3-5 minutes
  - Cut some onion into small pieces; add it to the pot
  - Wrap the pot in a towel to maintain the temperature for 15-30 minutes
  - Add some butter or vegetable oil before eating.

If you find buckwheat prepared this way difficult to digest, use the regular cooking method.

The principles of eating fats

Animal fats: butter, cream, grease, etc.
Plant oils: vegetable oil, various nuts, etc.

1. Fats can be combined with carbohydrates and vegetables.
2. Limit your daily fat intake to about 1oz (28g) of vegetable oil and 0.3-0.5oz (10-15g) of butter (2 tablespoons).

Some useful advice:

- Heating fats above 302F (150C) – the temperature in a frying pan – causes them to become particularly harmful. All fats, including vegetable oils, break up into toxic substances in such temperatures.
  When we fry in high temperature, the fried food forms a polyethylene-like lining. It contains carcinogenic substances – eating fried foods increases our risk of cancer and liver diseases.

106

It is best to use only unheated oils and add them to our meals shortly before eating.

- Many additives, especially preservatives, are used in the production of butter to extend its usefulness for a few months. It is a good idea to purify butter (remove additives) by melting it in water. Pure butter does not cause high cholesterol levels and can be stored for a long time without any preservatives.

Removing additives from butter

Put 9oz (250g) of butter in a pot, pour one cup (240ml) of warm boiled water over it and slowly boil for one hour. Then let it cool off, put it in the refrigerator, and pour the water out when the butter is solid.

All additives contained in butter are dissolved and are discarded with water during the process.

The principles of eating fruits

1. It is best to eat small amounts of fruits 20-30 minutes before meals.
2. Don't add sugar to raw fruits. Try to eat fruits in their natural ripening season. Fruits cleanse our blood (remove acids). When we add sugar, it causes the opposite effect.

The principles of eating vegetables

1. In the winter and spring it is better not to rely too much on tomatoes and cucumbers. These vegetables are artificially grown or harvested before they are ripe and start rotting soon after that. In order to extend their shelf life, they are treated with various substances. Everybody knows the harmful effects of such substances on our health.
2. Many people complain that eating raw vegetables causes them discomfort.
   It happens because they do not chew their vegetables well enough. All plant-based foods ought to be chewed thoroughly

– the digestion process starts in the mouth. If these foods are not chewed well, they ferment in the stomach, where they cause bloating and excess gas. (It is a good idea for people with more than four teeth missing to use a grater, preferably a plastic one, when preparing their vegetables).

3. Many vegetables contain traces of radioactive substances. If possible, we should grow our own vegetables or buy organically grown ones. If this is not possible, we can remove about 40% of the radioactive substances by soaking the vegetables in salty water in a dark place for three hours.

4. During the cold seasons, we can use pickled vegetables, dried fruits, and processed fruits as our sources of vitamins and microelements.

Some useful advice concerning fruits and vegetables:

It is best to eat fruits and vegetables that are locally grown and to eat them in their natural ripening season. Different climates cause the plants to contain different biological information.

Plants grown in hot climates develop cooling qualities in their juices. Melons, oranges, mandarins, and bananas cool off our body. If we live in the northern climates, we should not eat citrus fruits in large quantities in the wintertime. If our region produces strawberries, raspberries, apples, cherries, and pears in the summertime, these are the fruits best for us to eat. In the summer, we can dry carrots, parsley, apples, pears, apricots, and plums in the sunshine. They can be soaked in water (from melted ice) in the wintertime and added to our fruit and vegetable soups and to our grains. This way we preserve 100% vitamin content of our fruits or vegetables for the rest of the year.

Plants growing in colder climates have the opposite, warming, qualities. When we eat grains, nuts, sunflower seeds, pumpkin seeds and root crops, they have a warming effect. The conclusion is simple: **We should eat more fruits and vegetables in the summertime for their cooling effect; in the wintertime, grains and dried fruits will help us keep warm.**

All processes in our body are governed by the natural law of duality and opposing factors (left and right arm, left and right brain hemisphere, etc.). Two elements – sodium and potassium – have a very important function in our body. They regulate the body's water economy by influencing the exchange of fluids in different ways. The proportion of sodium (Na) to potassium (K) should be 1:20. If the balance is shifted either way, it interferes with our life processes. We should try to maintain the golden mean. **If you are swollen and feel excess of water in your body, eat products rich in potassium: peas and squash. In he opposite case – if you feel deficiency of water, eat more products that help retain water in you body: olive oil, pears, raspberries, blackcurrant, carrot, apples, apricots, tomatoes, millet, buckwheat, and oat. The perfect proportion of sodium and potassium is found in potatoes, cherries, cucumbers, and cabbage.**

In the summertime, the best kind of breakfast is one consisting of fruits. They are rich in all elements essential for our body, increase the alkalinity of our blood, provide plenty of energy, and do not use much energy to be digested.

How should we eat our desserts?

We usually eat desserts at the end of our main meals, when the stomach is already full. All deserts – cakes, ice cream, sweet fruits, candy, biscuits, etc. – make a very bad combination with other kinds of foods. When they get into our already full stomach, they slow down the digestive process. This way they cause fermentation in our digestive tract. The best advice is to avoid desserts or eat them separately.

If you are going to have a piece of cake, eat plenty of raw vegetables afterwards. Ice cream should not be combined with any other food – do not eat anything else for the next two to three hours.

Cold desserts (ice cream, sweet beverages) cool off our stomach's neighboring organs and reduce their blood supply, causing cramps. Enzymes used for digestion need temperatures above 98.6F (37C) to be active. Any cold food has to be warmed before it can be digested – this uses an extra amount of energy. Ice cream and cold beverages may be the cause of lumps and cysts in the case of females, and prostate inflammations in the case of males. It is better to consume them very infrequently and only in the hot seasons.

The secrets of healthy diet

Based on the position of the Sun, the ancients used a concept distinguishing three consecutive periods in a day. Each period lasts four hours. The cycle of three periods repeats itself so that each period occurs twice within 24 hours.

The first period (6a.m.-10a.m.) is the period of peace. The Sun is rising, the surroundings are peaceful, and our body begins to wake up. We are rested – there is no need for large amounts of energy. A large breakfast would put unnecessary strain on our body. It is enough to drink a glass of fruit or vegetable juice and eat one fruit or vegetable. Other types of foods take 1.5-2 hours before they yield their energy. For breakfast it is better to eat something easily absorbable that provides energy without taking much time to be digested. Fruits, vegetables, and their juices are the most appropriate foods.

The second period starts at 10a.m. and ends at 2p.m. The Sun is high in the sky. We feel hungry – our "digestive fire" is most intense (just as the heat of the Sun). We should eat our largest meal during this period (about 11a.m.-2p.m.). Starchy foods and vegetables would be the best combination. They provide large amounts of energy needed for the second half of the day.

The third period (2p.m.-6p.m.) is characterized by motion. The Sun heats up the air and the ground, and winds are stirred up. People become more active and work intensely, using up the energy acquired from the food.

Then the cycle of periods is repeated (6p.m.-10p.m.; 10p.m.-2a.m.; 2a.m.-6a.m.). Based on the biological rhythms, it is best to eat supper before sunset. The day is over and our body does not need much energy. Our "digestive fire" diminishes as the Sun goes down. It is the best time to eat protein foods because they need long and slow digestion (3-7 hours).

The best time to go to bed is before 10p.m. (before the second period is repeated). Otherwise we feel hungry again and gravitate towards the refrigerator. But our bodily organs also have a certain schedule. The digestive organs are active in the morning and the afternoon. In the evening and at night, excretory organs do their work.

This schedule is violated if we eat at night. The digestive organs take away some energy needed by excretory organs. Even then, digestion is incomplete and deposits of mucus, toxins, and fat

110

are formed. **Night eating is a sure way to cause kidney and liver stones, insomnia, weak immune system, and nervous disorders. Lack of regard for the laws of nature brings punishment in the form of weak vital functions and chronic diseases (heart disease, circulatory, liver, and kidney disorders).**

If we want to have a lot of energy for our daily activities, we should wake up in the third period (before 6a.m.) Waking up in the first period (6a.m.-10a.m.) causes us to feel tired and frustrated all day. Remember: The early bird gets the worm.

Scheduling your day in accordance with biological rhythms

Using the following advice will make you feel alert and energetic and will guarantee good health.

1. Get up between 5 a.m. and 6 a.m.
2. Rinse out your mouth.
3. Drink half a glass of spring water, mineral water, or water from melted ice with a teaspoon of honey.
4. Wash your face and brush your teeth.
5. Massage your ears by stretching and rubbing them with your hands for about one minute.
6. Perform any set of exercises strengthening your spine.
7. Massage your body with a moist, warm towel until your skin is red in color and then take a shower.
8. Your shower should be alternately hot and lukewarm, lukewarm and cool, hot and cold. Keep the temperatures within a comfortable range.
9. Pour some water (4-6 inches/10-15cm) in a basin; put in some rounded pebbles and walk in place on the pebbles (2-3 minutes) to massage your feet. Towel-dry your feet thoroughly and put on a pair of socks.
10. Perform cleansing breathing exercises for 2-4 minutes (see page 76).
11. Walk fast or jog (depending on your physical condition) 2-3 miles (3-5km), if possible in the woods or a park.
12. I personally prefer having two meals a day: one around noon and one between 6 p.m. and 7 p.m. This is especially better for people whose jobs are mostly intellectual in nature. For

those whose work involves more physical effort, the following meal schedule is recommended:
- Breakfast between 7 a.m. and 9 a.m.
- Lunch between 11 a.m. and 2 p.m.
- Supper between 6 p.m. and 8 p.m.

13. At 10 p.m. perform 10-15 cleansing breaths.
14. Take an alternate hot-cold shower.
15. Your sleep between 10 p.m. and 2 a.m. is very calm, deep, and restful (especially for your nervous system). If you cannot fall asleep between 10 p.m. and 11 p.m., but you go to sleep between 1 a.m. and 3 a.m., set your alarm at 5 a.m. for the first four days. You will feel tired in the first days, but it will allow you to set your sleep time in accordance with your physiology.

People whose daily schedule follows the just described pattern are in tune with the laws of nature and with their body's physiology.

How to plan a healthy diet

Most of us do not plan our diet in a systematic manner; we just want our food to be easily prepared, tasty, and plentiful. Our body is unable to properly digest the large volumes we eat, and to properly dispose of the waste. In spite of that, we keep putting strain on our body by taking in new loads of food.

The more we eat, the more often we feel hungry. Healthy appetite becomes replaced by permanent excessive hunger. We swell from too much fluids and salt; our bodies become rounded and shapeless. A large belly makes it hard to tie our shoestrings. The spine is bent out of shape under the weight of our body. Our heart is overworked and can hardly pump thick blood polluted with acids. With bitterness and regret, we watch our lazy, aggressive, and ill children and grandchildren. Our statistics boast about increased average longevity, yet many people do not live even half the number of years nature intended for them. If we want to explain all these negative phenomena, we have to look mainly at our bad nutritional habits.

In the recent years, research was done about the nutritional habits of our ancestors and the diseases they suffered from. The data show that, throughout most of our evolution, human beings ate mainly simple, plant-based foods.

An ancient cabalistic writing about the origins of dynasties and tribes contains an explanation of high longevity (500-700 years) enjoyed by people living before the Great Flood. The explanation is in their diet. They ate only foods yielded by the Earth and drank only pure water. After the Flood, Noah's children were allowed to eat meat and drink wine. This became the cause of a shorter life span. The constant progress of civilization completely changed our way of life since then, but our genes have not changed.

Empty calories

Contemporary nutritional science looks mainly at the calories obtained by our body from the food. Ancient dieticians were not interested just in the calories. They looked at both energy and biological information contained in the food and tried to understand how both factors influence our body. For example, the effects of eating an apple on a hot summer day are very different from the effects of eating it on a cold winter day, even though it contains the same amount of calories. Eating apples in the winter often causes chills, stomach pains and excessive gas. It cannot be explained by calorie content, but from the point of view of ancient dieticians it is easily explainable. The biological information contained in the apple is appropriate for the summer. It triggers mechanisms that keep our body moist and cool. The sweet or sour taste of an apple also has a cooling effect. According to ancient theories, each food product by means of its taste and color retains information about the place where it grows, about its temperature, humidity, etc. When we eat natural plant-based products, we can feel connected with the great wonders of nature. Foods obtained from plants always have unique color, taste, and aroma, unlike artificial foods created by men. The fundamental rule in our ancestors' diet was the following: **Eat foods grown in your region and in accordance with their natural ripening season, because that way you share in the might and wisdom of nature.** Our ancestors tried to understand the very essence of nutrition and used food as their medicine. Our understanding of nutrition, so important in sustaining our life, has been narrowed by contemporary science.

The principles of self-digestion

We are often intrigued by the fact that while eating the same kind of food, with the same amount of calories, some of us get fat and others do not. Some of us remain slim even if they eat pounds of sweets; others gain weight after having just one piece of chocolate. A dinner can be very nutritious for the mother, useless for the daughter, and outright harmful for the father's health. We get different results by consuming foods with the same amount of calories because each of us is a unique creature.

There is a system that can solve many nutritional problems – nutrition based on different nutritional types among people. It uses an analogy to what happens in nature: different kinds of animals eat different foods. Tigers get their nutrition from meat and rabbits from carrots (without peeling them). Even the form in which food enters the digestive tract is different for different animals. A python has to swallow a rabbit in one piece together with its fur; otherwise it would not be digested properly. People are divided into certain types based on their individual qualities. For each type, there is a group of food products that is best absorbed and most beneficial.

In nature there is a principle of self-digestion. Food (plant or animal) is digested in 50% by enzymes contained in its own tissue, not in the digestive juices of the eater. The digestive juices just trigger the mechanism of self-digestion.

Each natural product contains biological information, like a code or password. If our digestive system has the ability to read this code, we can digest the food product without using much energy.

We can use an analogy to Rubik's cube. If we know a code, we can solve the cube in a few seconds. Solving it without a code takes a lot of time and effort. Digestion in our body works in a similar manner. **Different types of people need different types of food. If we try to nurture our body with food that is inappropriate for us, we become weak and ill.**

Food of the wise

Based on the ability to absorb food, the ancients divided people into three types:
X (wind), Y (bile), and Z (mucus).

114

Type X physical characteristics:

1. Thin bones, slim figure, short or medium height, ill-looking, always cold, shy by nature
2. Slim hands, cold and dry in touch
3. Quick movements, light and smooth walk

Physiological qualities:

1. Steady body weight maintained without dieting, frequent digestive troubles
2. Shallow, short sleep

Psychological and intellectual qualities:

1. Cheerful, energetic
2. Quick absorption of information, short retention
3. Easy to socialize and communicate with

Preferred type of food:

Fatty and oily foods in large quantities

Seasons of the year:

1. Hot seasons preferred
2. Low tolerance for cold, dry skin in the winter

Typical health problems:

Dry skin, constipation, joint and bone pains

Most appropriate types of food:

1. Grains: rice, wheat, barley, corn, buckwheat
2. Dairy products: all kinds in moderation
3. Sugars: honey, raw sugar, jams
4. Vegetable oils: all kinds
5. Fruits: melons, other kinds of sweet fruits
6. Vegetables (raw): beets, carrot, asparagus, potatoes, cucumbers, onions
7. Nuts: all kinds

8. Animal products: beef, pork, fish, chicken, duck, rabbit, eggs
9. Seasoning: garlic, onion, ginger, cinnamon, black pepper, cumin, salt, mustard
10. Soups: nettle, garlic

Type Y physical characteristics:

1. Average body size, fine red or grey hair, balding
2. Average hand size, warm and pleasant in touch
3. Calm movements, normal, smooth walk

Physiological qualities:

1. Good digestion with regular meal times, otherwise irritable
2. Normal sleep, frequent dreams

Psychological and intellectual qualities:

1. Well organized and thorough
2. Different levels of mental capacity
3. Easily irritable

Preferred type of food:

Cool meals in moderate amounts

Seasons of the year:

Low tolerance for summer heat, easily fatigued on hot summer days; warm autumn, and warm rainy days preferred

Typical health problems:

Inflammations, fever, digestive system diseases, liver diseases, heartburn, agitation, and irritability

Most appropriate types of food:

1. Cool, usually liquid products, fluids (tea, mineral water, coffee)

2. Grains: wheat, oat, barley, wheat sprouts, rice, corn
3. Dairy products: butter
4. Sugars: all kinds except honey, in moderation
5. Oils: olive, sunflower, and corn
6. Fruits: melon, lemon, grapefruit, orange, other sweet fruits (fresh or dried)
7. Vegetables: pumpkin, cucumber, potatoes, cabbage, beans, peas, parsnips and parsley
8. Seasoning: coriander, cinnamon, black pepper, dill, occasionally garlic
9. Soups: vegetable
10. Animal products: beef, egg yolk, fish, lamb, seafood

Type Z physical characteristics:

1. Thick bones, tendency to be overweight
2. Big hands, cold and moist in touch
3. Slow, smooth movements; walk slow and heavy

Physiological qualities:

1. Slow physiological processes
2. Moderate eating, tendency to gain weight, difficult weight reduction
3. Calm sleep, at least eight hours a day required

Psychological and intellectual qualities:

1. Very cautious, every action carefully thought through
2. Easy absorption and retention of information
3. Peaceful and hard to irritate but once upset, persistent in the confrontation

Preferred type of food:

Warm, dry and low-fat foods in moderate amounts

Seasons of the year:

A dislike for rainy and humid weather (tendency to depression)

Typical health problems:

Obesity, depression, chills, pale skin, possible frequent colds

Most appropriate types of food:

1. Warm and light meals, herbal tea and mineral water to drink, all in moderation
2. Grains: barley, corn, millet, buckwheat, oat, rice
3. Dairy products: skim milk, fresh butter, aged cheese, cream, kefir
4. Sugars: honey
5. Vegetable oils: all kinds, especially corn oil
6. Fruits: apples, pears, pomegranates, grapes, quince, melons, moderation recommended with very sweet fruits
7. Vegetables: potatoes, carrots, cabbage, onion, tomatoes, turnip, green vegetables, pumpkin, celery, spinach, parsley, beans and peas
8. Seasoning: all kinds, not too much salt
9. Soups: vegetable soups, low fat meat soups
10. Animal products: chicken, eggs, beef, pork, lobster
11. Nuts: all kinds

Most people's characteristic is a combination of two types, but one of them always dominates and the other is represented in a weaker form. The division described here is just a generalization. It would be necessary to know a person's date, hour, and place of birth in order to prescribe individually the optimum diet. You can, however, get good results by using this general categorization while you plan your menu.

Some useful advice:

The ancients used a simple and easy method to predict whether a food product was appropriate for their body. They held the product in one hand and focused their mind on the question whether it was good for them, while in the other hand they held a golden ring hanging on a cotton thread about 30inches/80cm long). When the ring's motion formed a circle (either clockwise or counter-clockwise), the answer to the question was supposed to be positive. If the ring swayed to the sides and its movement did not form a circle, the food was considered inappropriate for that person. In some cases, the outcome for the same product changed after some time – it meant that the product was finally accepted by the body and was safe to eat. If the outcome was consistently negative after a few experiments, that food product was inappropriate for the particular person and was to be avoided entirely.

When you find a diet that is most appropriate, you will notice the following changes:

1. You will become more active both intellectually and physically.
2. Your hearing and sight will improve.
3. Your eyes will look clear.
4. The color of your tongue will be pink – white and grey layers will disappear.
5. The complexion of your face will look healthier.
6. Your nails and hair will grow better.

The taste of foods

There are only six tastes in the world of foods. The way we combine the tastes decides whether our meals bring us energy and health or excess fat and disease.

When we eat we do not think that different flavors affect our body in different ways. The flavors tell us about the qualities of energy contained in the food products. Our tongue, acting as the taste organ, allows us to identify these kinds of energy. There are six flavors: sweet, sour, salty, bitter, astringent, and pungent.

Sweet – Energizes the whole body; stimulates weight increase; used in excess stimulates the production of mucus and fat; reduces the body's ability to generate heat. People whose diet includes a lot of sweet-tasting products become lazy, dull and overweight. Sweet taste characterizes sugar, honey, milk, cream, wheat products, fruits, vegetables, beans, peas, nuts and sunflower seeds. Citrus fruits have sour and sweet tastes.

Sour – Has refreshing qualities, stimulates appetite, helps retain fluids in the body, improves intellectual abilities, regulates digestive processes. Excess worsens the blood composition, causes ulceration, skin irritation and heartburn. Too much sour taste in our food causes us to be overactive, irritable and short-tempered. Kefir and various cheeses are sour or pungent.

Salty – Has purifying qualities, removes mold, stimulates appetite, improves digestion, helps retain fluids, helps remove excessive mucus and stomach juices. Ancient Greeks used to suck on salt crystals after their meals and spit out the salty saliva. The word "salt" is derived from a word meaning "Sun" – the salty taste generates "digestive fire" in our body by stimulating the action of digestive enzymes. Salt gets into the blood stream together with the stomach juice and circulating in the body dissolves old, cancerous, and other diseased cells without damaging the healthy ones. Recent research shows that under the age of one our body contains only 1% old cells, at the age of 10 – 7% old cells, and at the age of 50 – 40% old cells. In other words, at the age of 50 our body is left with only 60% of its full capacity – the percentage of remaining young cells. To improve the balance in favor of young cells, we should eat salty foods of natural sources.

I recommend that, after each meal, you put 2-3 salt crystals on your tongue, suck on them, and then spit out the saliva.

Bitter – Improves appetite and digestion, warms up the body, stimulates the removal of fluids, cleanses the body and dilutes blood. The consumption of bitter foods helps in body cleansing and weight reduction. Excess of bitter taste causes loss of strength, stimulates anxiety and fear. Roasted seeds, lemon peel, cucumbers, and some other vegetables are bitter in taste.

Astringent – Has drying qualities, helps to heal wounds by drying pus and blood, improves skin complexion. Green-leafed vegetables, pears, cabbage, potatoes are examples of astringent-tasting products.

Pungent – Normalizes the functioning of the gastrointestinal tract, improves appetite. Pungent taste is represented by foods such as onion, garlic, chili pepper, radish, turnips, and spices. Kefir and various cheeses are sour or pungent.

We can influence many processes taking place in our body by skillfully combining food flavors in our meals.

If we constantly feel cold, we should eat meals containing bitter and sour tastes. This combination causes our body to warm up and stimulates weight loss. Combining sour and salty flavors produces the warming effect but also causes weight gain. The combinations of sweet with salty or sweet with sour flavors also stimulate weight gain – we gain fat in the first case and muscle mass in the second. Meals combining bitter and astringent tastes make us more energetic. They increase our mobility and physical fitness and are recommended for people with low blood pressure and poor circulation.

The huge variety of food products makes it impossible to categorize everything. We all have an intuitive understanding of basic taste categories.

Product tastes

Each type of taste stimulates a specific organ in our body: sour taste – the liver, salty – the kidneys, bitter – the heart, sweet –pancreas, pungent – the lungs, and astringent – the large intestine.

People who enjoy good health should eat food products that include all six tastes, without overusing any of them. Such diet harmoniously stimulates our body's energy. Those who need to suppress weight gain can do it by skillfully combining tastes in their meals. The world of tastes is very interesting and extensive. Discussing it fully would require a separate book. The following short section on tastes can only serve to stimulate some people's curiosity and show how much there is still to know about food – a subject each of us deals with every day.

The digestive fire

In ancient times, root spices were worth their weight in gold. Small amounts of them were added to food in order to improve the functioning of the digestive system, making digestion a few times easier.

Our ability to digest food becomes weaker as we age. As adults, we like to talk about how we were able to eat everything when we were younger. Now we often experience troubles in our stomach, intestinal disorders, and the sensation of heaviness in our whole body.

According to Eastern wisdom, poor digestion is the main source of diseases. The concept of digestive fire is used in the East to explain this relationship. If the fire is strong and bright (as in our young years), food is digested well, without toxic remains. The cells receive necessary nourishment and our body is healthy. When the digestive fire becomes weak with age, digestion is incomplete and toxins are formed, putting us at risk of all types of diseases. To revitalize the weakening digestive fire, we can add the following products to our meals: black or red pepper, cardamom, cinnamon, cloves, mustard, horseradish, ginger, and salt.

By taking small amounts of these products before, during, or after our meals, we can stimulate our appetite or improve our body's digestive function. We especially need spices during cold seasons. The elderly people and others with weak digestion can benefit greatly from adding spices to their food. We should all add some ginger to our meals and tea to revitalize our digestion. **Ginger is regarded in the East to be the best product able to rebuild our body's digestive powers.**

Ginger therapy

Ancient dieticians recommended a special ginger therapy to improve digestion. The therapy is intended for older people, whose digestive fire naturally diminished with age. It is not recommended for the young and middle-aged whose digestive disorders have other causes.

Preparation: Take a small enamel or ceramic bowl; mix four tablespoons of powdered ginger with 3.6-5.4oz (100-150g) of melted butter, and stir until you get a uniform blend. Cover it with a lid and keep in a cool place.

Take the mixture before breakfast everyday. The breakfast should consist of herbal tea, freshly steamed vegetables and grains

- Day 1 – half a teaspoon
- Day 2 – 1 teaspoon
- Day 3 – 1.5 teaspoons
- Day 4 – 2 teaspoons
- Day 5 – 2.5 teaspoons
- Day 6 – 2.5 teaspoons
- Day 7 – 2 teaspoons
- Day 8 – 1.5 teaspoons
- Day 9 – 1 teaspoon
- Day 10 – half a teaspoon

As we can see, the amount increases by half a teaspoon a day, then levels out, and then starts decreasing on day 7. The amount on day 10 is half a teaspoon, same as on day 1.

When the therapy is ended, our digestive fire will be revitalized. During the therapy we are to avoid products with strong cooling qualities, such as ice water, ice cream, refrigerated milk, frozen fruits or berries, etc.

Melting butter to improve its qualities. Melt regular butter on a frying pan using low heat until it becomes thick and has an olive color and then cool it off. Butter prepared this way is clean of additives, does not increase cholesterol levels, and can be stored for a long time without any preservatives.

How much should we eat?

My answer to this question is: the less the better! Nobody dies of moderation. People get ill and die because of overeating.

The capacity of a normal human stomach is 12-15 fl oz (350-450ml). However, most people's stomach is stretched to an unnatural size and they eat five to ten times the amounts their body really needs. It is a serious mistake to get into the habit of overeating; we should resist it just like any other bad habit.

We should follow Hippocrates' advice: **"If you still have a slight sensation of hunger after a meal – you have eaten well. If you feel full – you have poisoned yourself."** If we put our palms together and curve our fingers, the space enclosed by the palms represents approximately the capacity of our stomach. A meal should not be bigger than half of this space. The amount of fluids consumed at a time should not fill more than a quarter of the space. The remaining quarter is needed to hold air. This is all that our stomach is designed to accommodate. If we consume meals larger than our stomach's physiological capacity day after day, the stomach becomes gradually stretched.

People with unnaturally stretched stomachs experience constant hunger and the more they eat the more food it takes for them to feel full. To break this vicious circle, they need to get out of the habit of eating fast – it is simple but very useful advice: eat slowly and chew your food very thoroughly.

123

The golden mean

The food we eat makes our blood acidic or alkaline. People in good health have blood that is 60-70% alkaline. A lower alkalinity factor (50-60%) is characteristic for people who often get different diseases. Acidic blood flows in the veins of chronically ill people. The following proportion of food groups in our daily diet promotes our bloods alkalinity:

- 60% fruits and vegetables
- 20% proteins
- 14% carbohydrates
- 6% fats

This kind of diet promotes the alkalinity of our blood and the acidity of other bodily fluids. Acidic bodily fluids make it impossible for disease-causing bacteria to develop and they also prevent putrefaction, fermentation, the formation of mucus and other unhealthy deposits. Our meals should make us feel light, energetic, and refreshed. If we feel sleepy and heavy in the stomach, if we experience gas or other unpleasant consequences, the type of food we eat is not appropriate for us or the amount is too large.

Changing eating habits

In our eating habits, we often neglect the principles by which our body works. Our body tries to follow the rules given by nature, but we teach it laziness and overeating. This conflict maintains our body in a half-diseased state. At last our body gives in and becomes chronically ill.

Let's try to find a better way to nurture our body, which would reward us with energy, strength, a refreshed spirit, and a clear mind.

It is best to introduce the changes gradually:

1. Start drinking vegetable juices (a glass twice a day) without changing the rest of your diet (1-1.5 months).
2. Add more vegetables to your diet. Fresh, steamed, and cooked vegetables should represent 30-40% of your menu (1.5-2 months).
3. Make changes in favor of raw food products (roughly 60% raw – 40% cooked).

4. Eat mostly plant-based foods and other products such as honey, eggs, plain yogurt, kefir, and cottage cheese. Drink herbal tea and freshly squeezed fruit and vegetable juices.
5. Arrange your meals in the correct order: fluids 20 minutes before any solid food, fruits before other foods, vegetable salads with carbohydrates (grains, potatoes, etc.) or with protein foods (fish, peas, eggs).
6. Limit artificially grown, refined, and smoked products to a minimum.

Let us summarize now all principles of a healthy diet. Practicing these principles will definitely improve your health.

The principles of a healthy diet:

1. Eat food products grown in your geographical region.
2. Eat fruits, vegetables, and nuts strictly in their natural ripening season.
3. Each meal should include raw (summer), steamed or pickled (winter) vegetables.
4. Try to eat yeast free breads and whole-grain baked goods.
5. In combining food products, follow the rules in Table 2 (page 103).
6. Chew your food thoroughly (30 to 50 times each bite).
7. Prepare your food directly before your meals.
8. Do not keep any leftovers to be later warmed up and eaten.
9. Reduce the amount of foods with artificial ingredients, refined foods, and smoked products.
10. Avoid eating instant meals and canned food products as much as possible.
11. Limit your intake of coffee and tea.
12. Add spices such as pepper and ginger to your foods (especially in the winter).
13. In the summer and fall, make some days "strawberry only," "cherry only," "apple only," or "watermelon only" days.
14. Fast once a week for 16 or 24 hours – during that time drink only boiled water.
15. When carrots, beets, or apples are in season, drink freshly squeezed juices (about 33 ounces / 1L a day).

16. Prevent constipation – it is the main enemy of your health and the main cause of aging.
17. Use moderation in your eating Monday through Friday.
18. Make Saturday and Sunday your feast days and eat everything you crave for. This advice does not really contradict the principles of healthy eating. According to the ancient doctors, even poison in small amounts can serve as a medication.

Our diet and cancer

The great Hippocrates liked to say that food should be our medicine.

According to the American Cancer Institute data, improper diet causes 40% of cancers in men and 60% in women. Carcinogenic substances in our food act slowly, but they systematically poison our body day by day.

There is more and more information available about the connection between our food and cancer. It turns out that our diet can cause cancer or alternatively protect us against it. The word "prevention" might seem overused. However, there is never too much emphasis on prevention if it can save us many years of treatment. Everybody should realize that our diet might become the cause of cancer.

Use two basic rules in your diet to make sure it is cancer preventing and not cancer-causing:

1. Avoid certain ingredients that can cause malignant tumors.
2. Include in your diet foods that contain substances protecting your body from cancer.

Let me explain these two rules:

Ingredients that can cause malignant tumors

Beware of fat!
Fats in our diet can be a source of carcinogenic substances. Old and used fats are many times more dangerous than fresh ones. **Never leave grease in your frying pan for a later use. If possible, replace fried meals with cooked and baked ones. It is a good idea to cut as much**

fat out of meat as possible. **Also limit your consumption to about two tablespoons a day.**

Smoked food products are particularly dangerous for our health because smoke deposits harmful compounds in them, including carcinogenic ones. Such compounds have been detected in smoked sausage, ham, bacon, and fish as well as in fruits dried with the use of smoke. Harmful substances contained in 1.8oz (50g) of smoked sausage may cause as much damage to our health as one pack of cigarettes or four days' worth of breathing polluted city air.

Health-damaging chemical compounds

Many food products contain nitrates and nitrites. These salts are not carcinogenic themselves, but in the process of digestion in our stomach, they can be turned into very harmful substances. Nitrates and nitrites can be found in sausages, some canned meats, and some store-bought fruits and vegetables. **This is why it is best to eat vegetables grown in the open air (not in a greenhouse!) with the use of natural fertilizers (e.g. compost).** If you cook vegetables, use plenty of water. Discard the water if you are not sure how the vegetables were grown.

Bigger belly – bigger problems

When a scientist from Philadelphia was asked if he knew a good diet to prevent cancer, he said: "Yes! You just have to eat less." Most experts agree with this opinion. **Research involving large population samples proves that obesity significantly increases the likelihood of cancer.**

How can we moderate our appetite? We can do it by eating aged breads, beans, peas, roasted sunflower seeds, and grains.

The sensation of hunger is often confused with the sensation of thirst. If we try drinking slowly a glass or two of water instead of having something to eat, the sensation of hunger often goes away after ten to fifteen minutes.

Substances that protect us from cancer

Our diet should contain ingredients that improve our immune system and help it protect us from the effects of carcinogenic substances and other harmful compounds. These healthy ingredients are, first of all, vitamins.

The connection between vitamins and our health is common knowledge. There is no need here to get into much detail about benefits coming from vitamins. I would only like to mention a few of them that are most important in cancer prevention. These are vitamins A, C, and E.

Vitamin A

The main role of vitamin A is programming a number of chemical reactions that protect us from different forms of cancer. Vitamin A is synthesized from beta-carotene in our digestive tract, where the vitamin is absorbed. The process takes place with the help of bile. If there are irregularities in the function of the digestive system, the liver, or the gallbladder, the amount of absorbed vitamin A is inadequate. It is a case of hidden deficiency in vitamin A. We are convinced that our food provides enough vitamin, but in reality not enough of it is absorbed, and our body experiences deficiency.

This is why it is very important to have our liver (which is our body's chemical laboratory) and our digestive system (especially the large intestine) in a perfect working order.

Animal liver and liver oil are very rich in vitamin A. It is also found in smaller concentrations in eggs, butter, and other milk products. Carotene, which turns into vitamin A in our body, is contained in carrots, red peppers, parsley, spinach, onion, apricots, tomatoes, pumpkin, and other fruits that are yellowish-red, or orange in color.

There is a simple test for vitamin A deficiency. Walk quickly from a well-lit room into a dark room. If in a few seconds you can distinguish shapes of things in the dark room, your body has an adequate amount of vitamin A. If you cannot see any shapes for a longer time, you are vitamin A deficient. In this case, I would recommend drinking freshly squeezed carrot juice and beet juice (see juices, page 83).

Vitamin C

High content of vitamin C prevents nitrates and nitrites from turning into carcinogenic compounds.

Vitamin C promotes good absorption of iron in the intestinal tract.

Note: Some women suffer from very high menstrual flow. It is a likely sign of iron deficiency (anemia), especially if they smoke and do not eat enough vegetables. Vitamin C is the "fuse" of the flexibility and strength of our blood vessels.

Easy bruising is another symptom of vitamin C deficiency. Vitamin C is one of the substances necessary for the removal of bad cholesterol from our body. Those who enjoy a fat meal should eat a big plate of vegetable salad with each steak they have (three to five times larger in volume than the steak). If they do not stick to this rule, sooner or later they are going to suffer from serious health problems. Vitamin C is almost non-existent in animal-based food products.

The main sources of vitamin C (ascorbic acid) are fruits, vegetables, berries, and greens. The richest among them are wild rose fruit, black currant, red currant, horseradish, dill, and onion. Citrus fruits and apples also have high vitamin C content.

In the winter, we can get our vitamin C from potatoes, cabbage, sauerkraut, garlic, onion, citrus fruits and juices, dried fruits, and jams with low sugar content.

Vitamin E

Vitamin E is called "the elixir of youth" because it slows the aging of cells in our body and, at the same time, protects us from harmful products of fat oxidation. When fats are oxidized, toxic compounds are produced and have to be neutralized. If there is a shortage of vitamin E and these substances are not neutralized, they cause rigidity of our nerve tissue, blood vessels, and muscles.

Vitamin E deficiency is particularly dangerous for infants – it can result in leukemia, as well as sight and respiratory disorders.

They have a low concentration of vitamin E at birth. This deficiency is supposed to be supplemented by breast milk.

Cow's milk contains very limited amounts of vitamin E – many times smaller than woman's milk. This is another significant argument in favor of breast-feeding.

It is a very disturbing fact that in the recent years more cases of blood cancers among little children are diagnosed. I am strongly convinced that the main cause of these diseases is artificial food low in vitamin E.

Foods containing the most vitamin E are: calf liver, egg yolk, wheat, oats, rye, corn, peas, parsley, carrot, onion, and garlic.

Fibers

Physicians noticed that colon cancer, so common in Europe, is hardly ever found among the African population. They attributed it to the fact that their diet contains large amounts of natural products. Fiber contained in these foods works as sort of a "broom" in our intestines, quickly removing toxins, stopping rotting processes, and preventing harmful bacteria from producing carcinogenic substances. This is why I advise to start meals with vegetable salads. The main sources of fiber are wholegrain flour, breads, buckwheat, oat, and leafy vegetables.

Mineral salts containing magnesium, calcium and selenium are important in cancer prevention. Podded plants (beans, peas), wheat, rye, oats, buckwheat, fruits, and vegetables are rich in magnesium. Calcium is found in large amounts in poppy seeds, beans, carrot, cabbage, and cheese. Peas and beets are the richest in selenium.

Some data suggest that **mushrooms** (e.g. boletus) and **soy products** contain substances protecting us from cancer.

We should remember that no diet provides full protection against cancer, but the probability of getting the illness can be significantly reduced. A good variety of natural foods in our menu makes it possible for our body to find substances needed for healing.

Some oncologists maintain that cancer is our body's vengeance for improperly eaten meals. In 99% of the cases we invite cancer by poisoning ourselves, only 1% is caused by spontaneous changes in our body. This means that we are 1% victims and 99% authors of cancer.

What should we eat? What is a good diet? These are very interesting and, at the same time, very difficult questions.

MIND

What is a disease?

(The following segment does not apply to genetic diseases.)

There are volumes of medical books about diseases; millions of doctors and scientists try to explore their mysteries. Nobody is able to provide answers about the origin of diseases, probably because diseases as such do not have their own existence. What we call a disease is our body's reaction to something that interferes with its normal functioning. An organ remains ill, and is eventually destroyed, as long as the source of interference is not removed. A malfunctioning organ can negatively influence other organs and systems (circulatory, nervous, lymphatic) cooperating with it. There is constant struggle between health and illness in the life of our body. We could not stay alive without this struggle. In the case of common cold, for example, we may suffer from fever, headaches, bone aches, and general body weakness. Can we regard these as symptoms as a disease? Certainly, but high body temperature kills the disease-causing bacteria; mucus released by our body carries away toxins, while headaches, bone aches, and the feeling of weakness are side effects of our body's struggle to return to health.

What we call a disease is the defensive reaction of our body's mechanisms designed to maintain us healthy. We all have these mechanisms. They are necessary to remove disorders in the way our body functions. They also give us warning signals when these disorders begin.

To stay healthy, we need to listen and understand what our body is trying to communicate to us. Do not treat diseases as your worst enemy. In a sense, they force us to make the first step on the way towards a healthy lifestyle.

My journey to health was not easy. I was a very ill child, spending probably about 200 days out of the year in bed, fighting various infections and viruses. My mother was an emergency physician, very absorbed by her work, and she did not have much time to sit at my bedside. When I had a fever, she would give me a few strong doses of penicillin (very widely used in the sixties) to reduce the temperature. The fever was gone in a few days but my nose was plugged with mucus and my throat inflamed, red as a tomato. This meant for my mother the necessity of more radical measures. My tonsils were removed. This caused further complications – an inflammation in the maxillary sinus and partial loss of my sense of smell. Long and ineffective treatment of these complications with large doses of medications caused pain in the liver area. I also had allergic rashes on my hands, abdomen, and back. In addition, my diet was fat and sweet. No wonder I suffered from chronic pains under my right lowest rib. Frequent headaches had to be treated with painkillers. One day I became sick at school, and then I fainted. The school nurse contacted my mother, who suspected probable acute inflammation of appendix and made sure I was quickly brought to the surgical ward. Three hours later I was on the operating table and the head doctor of the surgical ward, a friend of my mother's, was operating on me. As it turned out, my appendix was perfectly healthy but my liver was enlarged and inflamed. The surgeon understood the source of my sufferings when she looked at my liver, but since my abdomen was already open, she removed my healthy appendix just in case. At least it was clear from now on that the cause of my headaches, weakness, and acute pain under the right lowest rib was my ill liver. Even though the appendix operation was successful, it caused complications in the form of hemorrhoids that afflicted me for many years.

As a result of such "close contact" with medicine, I gained a certain kind of experience. I understood that whenever medicine heals something in my body, it hurts (sometimes unknowingly) something else at the same time. When I later started helping other ill people, I was finally convinced that all pharmaceutical remedies could only maintain our body in a semi-healthy state. This is why a diagnosis so often has the word "chronic" in it (chronie inflammation of gallbladder, joints, etc.). Because "chronic" means "continual" and "unending," we can conclude that our diseases need to be treated for the rest of our lives.

Avicenna, Persian philosopher and physician, over 1000 years ago said:

A physician should have three things in his arsenal – words, medications, and a blade.

Words are necessary to explain to patients what mistakes they make in their lifestyle, and what is the connection between the mistakes and the source of illness.

Medications when words cannot explain the cause of the disease but there is still a duty to provide relief from suffering.

The blade is used when the physician cannot identify the source of the disease, influence the patient with words, or find any medication to reduce the pain. By using a surgical blade, the doctor only removes the effects of a well-advanced disease. Its source remains and is ready to manifest in new places. An operation usually provides only some temporary relief for the patients before they are afflicted with an even worse disease.

My experience taught me that the decisive factor in all matters of illness and health is the amount of energy available for our bodily organs. If there are deficiencies in the energy system that invisibly connects all our internal organs, our body becomes ill. Kan Funajana, an ancient Japanese physician, in his book "Guidelines of Medicine" wrote:

A human being is an entity whose soul and body form a union. This is why it is not possible to heal the body without considering the state of the soul and vice versa.

We already know that to maintain our body in good health we need to cleanse it regularly, nurture it properly, and build up its immunity with the use of water, fresh air, sunlight, and physical exercise. When we talk about the soul, we should think about the human bio-energy system. Our consciousness, feelings, and memories are forms of invisible energy about whose qualities we know very little. To regulate psychological processes, we need to learn their mechanisms and this involves learning about bio-energy.

Contemporary psychology considers only an insignificant number of bio-energetic processes taking place in our body. As far as medicine is concerned, it is mainly oriented towards treating the body and acknowledges little connection between the body and the soul. Our medicine focuses so much on different parts of the body that it almost forgets its existence as an integrated system.

I am convinced that as long as medicine will use this approach to the functioning of the human body, diseases will always remain chronic and incurable. Improved methods of treating effects are not going to remove causes and bring health. Medicine looks for answers dealing with more effective and painless methods of removing ill organs and uses constantly improving hardware. The very thought of pain caused by a low-speed dental drill used years ago makes everybody tremble. Today's high-speed drills and effective anesthetics make a dental procedure relatively painless for the patient. However, tooth decay and gum disease still exist and will continue to exist.

Contemporary methods allow a surgeon to remove the gallbladder in 30 minutes and use only a local anesthetic. A few years later the procedure brings effects in the form of digestive disorders.

A bypass surgery uses arteries or veins from other parts of the body to take over the role of a useless coronary artery in the circulatory system. The artery or vein to be grafted is taken from the same ill body and is only a little better - five or six years later, another bypass surgery will be required.

There are thousands of such examples. In my opinion, even perfectly successful surgeries in the long run are as ineffective as patching up an old pair of pants that are falling apart. A new patch in one place creates a tear in another and eventually the whole garment is beyond repair. People who are caught in these kinds of situations with their health problems would probably agree with me. Despite huge amounts of time spent on different treatments, their health does not improve. Are there solutions for such situations? I think there are.

We should work on creating a completely new approach to the question of healing our body:

1. Quit blaming our doctors for treating us ineffectively.
2. Understand that we are first to be responsible for taking care of our health.

We can learn to stop headaches by simple methods removing their causes instead of taking painkillers that poison our liver and our whole body. If the gallbladder is plugged up with stones, it needs to be cleansed, not removed. Heart disease, circulatory disorders, and obesity are results of laziness and lack of exercise. Pains in our stomach and pancreas come from overeating and not caring enough about providing the proper kind of nutrition for our body. I would like to be correctly understood – I am not advocating self-treatment.

Doctors have been, are, and will continue to be needed. We could not manage without them in extreme cases (e.g. accidents). However, we should also know how to take care of our body and help ourselves from day to day. We could use doctors only as our wise advisors.

Everybody, not only a group of trained professionals, can possess the knowledge necessary to maintain good health. We need to stay healthy in order to fully use our natural gifts such as intellect, strength, and goodness.

To be healthy, we should use the following principle of Hippocrates: "If you are not your own doctor, you are a fool."

The most important fact to remember, especially for those who need to recover their lost health, is that our organism is an integrated system and we have to treat it in a complex manner – both our body

134

and mind. Only this kind of approach brings results. Health involves striving for physical and spiritual perfection.

There is one more point I would like to make – we start causing damage to our health in various ways from early childhood. This is why we cannot expect an immediate return to health. It may take two to three years of work before we get rid of our health problems. Once we put our body and mind in order, we only need to persist in maintaining it and enjoy good health – a free gift from nature – for the rest of our life.

Learn about yourself

Seneca, a Roman philosopher, said: **"People do not die – they kill themselves."**

This brilliant statement is two thousand years old and we still resist the wisdom contained in it. I wonder why? Did not Seneca say it loud enough, or maybe people do not have enough time to take notice? In either case, we pass our bad habits from generation to generation, and along with the habits, we pass down diseases. As an excuse, we say that times are hard and the progress of civilization puts a heavy burden on us. However, we are rather burdened by our excess weight, laziness, and complete disregard for the physiological rules by which our body functions. We know how to deal with complicated economical problems, use computers, or repair an electronic instrument with thousands of connections, but we cannot answer the simple question about the number of times we urinate in a day or the color of our urine. I would like to stress: if we do not learn to watch how our body functions, we cannot maintain good health.

One day, while in a cafeteria, I saw a young woman with a troubled look on her face. She pulled some pills out of her purse and took one of them.

"What is troubling you?" – I asked.

She tried to smile friendly and answered in a tired voice.

"I have a headache again."

I looked more closely. Her eyes looked tired and slightly red. She had dark spots, freckles, moles, and lesions on her skin. The complexion on her face was yellowish-brown as it is usually in the case of female smokers. Despite her relatively young age

(25-27), she had rings under her eyes, deep wrinkle between the eyebrows, slightly swollen eyelids, and wilted skin on her neck and under her chin. Her back was bent and her neck had a limited range of motion.

"You work in an office, don't you?"

"How do you know?"

"Everyone who spends time at the desk suffers from headaches, low blood pressure, kidney diseases, and disorders of the reproductive organs. It is especially true for women. Your position at work is the cause of all these symptoms. Would you like to know what causes freckles, moles, and lesions on your skin?"

"Tell me – she said surprised."

"You have a misaligned spine and an ill liver. This causes skin spots and headaches. Please take a close look at your shoes."

Surprised, she pulled her feet from under the table.

"Your shoes are worn out in the front and the middle. It means your liver is ill."

"I don't understand what my shoes can tell you about my illnesses"

"They tell me a lot. The way they are wearing out signals diseases long before they are manifested in any other way. Ancient physicians discovered a close relationship between the condition of feet and the disorders of internal organs, such as liver or heart, which cause weakness in the legs. We start walking differently and wearing out our shoes in a very specific way. If the sole wears out quickly at the heel, it signals a kidney disorder. A worn tip and outer edges mean a heart disease. In your case, there is an indication of an ill liver. A malfunctioning liver results in poor blood filtering. Polluted blood circulates in the body and causes healthy organs to malfunction. There is a close connection between the liver and the skin. Dark spots, freckles, pimples, moles, or lesions are results of a poorly functioning liver."

"This is interesting" – she said with disbelief. Then she took another sip of coffee and was ready to listen again.

"How many cups of coffee have you had today?"

"Three or four. I have low blood pressure and frequently get headaches. Without a coffee, I feel sleepy."

"I can tell you why. Your kidneys don't function very well and this is, among others, the cause of low blood pressure. Coffee makes you feel alert for only 15-20 minutes and then you feel sleepy and tired again. Excessive amounts of coffee flush out very important elements such as iron, magnesium, and calcium from your body. Cigarettes that often go together with coffee cause vitamin C deficiency. You would have to drink juice squeezed from one lemon or orange after every cigarette to replenish the amount of vitamin C you lose. If you don't do it, you will eventually have dark rings under your eyes – one of the signs of anemia. Broken blood vessels, especially on your face and legs, mean deficiency in vitamin C and magnesium. I noticed that you like to have a sandwich and coffee to satisfy your hunger."

"That's right" – she admitted. "Coffee reduces my appetite."

"I disagree with that. Coffee is simply a stimulator. It gives you energy for a very short time, that's all. The habit of satisfying your hunger with a small sandwich leads to frequent constipation because a low-volume meal does not contain enough fiber to make our digestive tract, particularly our large intestine, work. Constipation causes self-poisoning in our body when food remains putrefied and toxins released by bacteria in the intestines are absorbed into the blood stream. These toxins are the cause of constant fatigue, headaches, insomnia, and nervous breakdowns."

"I admit that sometimes one pill is not enough to deal with a persistent headache" – she said and swallowed another pill.

"Why do you poison yourself? Every pill is a poison! Even if it stops your headache today, what are you going to do tomorrow or in a month? Will you just keep poisoning you body this way?"

"And what else can I do?"

"There are many ways to stop a headache without pills. Cover your forehead with your right hand; press the palm hard against the forehead and turn your head right 20 times, rubbing the forehead against the palm. Then repeat the same using your left hand. After that, use your thumbs and index fingers to massage your earlobes for 3-5 minutes. Massage hard – to the point of pain. You can do it now."

The entire uncomplicated procedure took her about five minutes. I asked her:

"How are you feeling now?"

"It stopped" – she said with disbelief. "What else can you tell me about my health?"

"You have a runny nose and breathe through your mouth. This is why you frequently have a sore throat, bronchi, and sore lungs. All these troubles are caused by your habit of sleeping on a soft mattress and a soft pillow."

The lady had her eyes wide open with surprise.

"It is sad that, at my age, I know so little about my body." – She looked slightly embarrassed. – "Please tell me what I should do."

"Change your lifestyle. Most of all, prevent constipation, improve the functioning of your intestines and liver, and finally put your spine in order. Start eating what is healthy and not what you like. Finally, understand one important truth – your health is in your own hands."

The healing thought

Self-healing method

Nature provided each one of us with an excellent individual "pharmacy" containing medicine against all diseases we can ever get. Our only task is learning how to make use of it.

The self-healing process has two stages. The first stage is to relax all the muscles in our body. In the second stage, we launch a healing program in our subconscious mind (just like a computer program) designed to trigger our body's self-regulatory processes. Self-healing is effective because it uses our body's natural defense mechanisms.

Stage 1 – relaxing

Spread a soft blanket on the floor and lie on your back. Your arms should be stretched alongside your body with the palms facing outside and the fingers slightly bowed, your feet tilted outside, your head turned to one side, mouth open, tongue against the upper teeth, and your eyes closed for better concentration. Try to be calm, not to think about anything, and, most important of all, breathe calmly and evenly. It usually takes two to five minutes to achieve full relaxation state.

Stage 2 – self-healing

The cells in our body have a basic mental capability similar to that of a little child. We should remember that fact when we address the ill organ. In your imagination try to visualize the malfunctioning organ, open communication with it, and concentrate on giving it an order. The order must be expressed clearly and decisively, as if you were trying to correct the behavior of your beloved child. Each one of our organs has its own "personality," for example our stomach and our liver are stubborn and not very reasonable. They need to be addressed in the form of a harsh command. Our heart is much wiser and it listens to requests expressed gently and cordially.

Having completed the first stage you can, for example, imagine looking inside your heart and try to see a small bright flame in it – the source of love and saving energy. Imagine that the flame grows, fills your whole heart, and then spreads throughout the entire body from the top of your head to the tips of your fingers and toes. Try to feel how it cleanses your body, removes inflammations, and brings health and vigor. Quietly say to yourself: "Every breath brings me closer to full cleansing. The light in my body is the healing energy." If you know a specific spot with a lump or inflammation, put your right hand on it and imagine that the healing light is emitted from the centre of your palm and it melts the lump just like sunrays melt snow or ice in the spring.

This was just an example. Everybody has enough imagination to develop his or her own healing scenario. The most important thing to remember is to relax your muscles and to enter the healing program into your subconscious mind. You can pick any time for self-healing sessions but it is better done when there is nobody around to interrupt you. If you enjoy quiet music, turn on your favorite piece for a better relaxation effect.

We can influence all our malfunctioning organs and systems, such as the nervous system, memory, vision, hearing, etc. in this manner. The method requires a serious approach and some acknowledgement from us that we are responsible for some of our health problems.

Positive attitude towards life

Death is not as terrifying as old age
— **Eastern wisdom**

Joyful old age

Throughout ages, people dreamed about being immortal and searched for the legendary elixir of youth. Many scientists in the world look for ways to extend the human life.

There are many who believe that we should not try to resist the aging process. They say that it is as pointless as trying to revive an old dying tree or renovate an old wooden house whose walls are falling apart. According to this view, all we can do is to influence the process of aging in a limited way by reducing the symptoms and preventing extreme suffering as the nature takes its course.

Then, why does the body age? One of the reasons is our own attitude that conditions the body to speed up the process.

We fear illness, immobility, and helplessness that come with the old age. Our aging process begins when we start dwelling on such thoughts and fears.

The way our aging process progresses greatly depends on our psychological attitude towards aging and death.

Unlike all other living organisms, we are able to influence all life processes in our body by using our mind. There are countless examples of people who became ill with a disease as a result of being preoccupied with fearful thoughts about it. There are just as many examples of individuals who conquered terminal diseases by maintaining a positive mental attitude.

Our thoughts have the power to make us healthy or ill; they can also make us younger or older.

Aging is the matter of attitude

When we start reflecting on our age, we usually think in terms of different milestones and stages of life: getting married, bringing up children, menopause for women, retirement, and so on. When we are strongly convinced that there is nothing we can do about the natural progression of the aging process, we program ourselves for premature aging. As soon as we notice our first wrinkles, the thinning of our hair, or pain in our joints, we pronounce the diagnosis: "I am getting old." We think that it creates the necessity to become less active, conserve energy, and lead a restful life. It does not occur to us that we brought these signs of aging on ourselves by incorrect diet, laziness, and lack of youthful enthusiasm for life. **We shorten our life ourselves by incorrectly using our psychological powers. Our aging process gets under way because we subconsciously anticipate it.**

The crucial period is the age between 40 and 50. During that period, we should pay particular attention to our hygiene and the condition of our skin, hair, hands, feet, and nails, to the flexibility and strength of our joints and muscles and to the overall shape of our body. Easy movements, straight posture, flexibility, flat abdomen, clear and bright eyes are the physical qualities of people who are not affected by aging. It is a mistake, especially for women, to avoid their image in the mirror as soon as they notice the first wrinkles on their face or fatty folds on their skin. Even though they try not to look in the mirror, they are subconsciously troubled by questions such as: "Is this really me? Has life worn me out so much? Do I look awful? Am I already getting old?"

Such concerns take away our enthusiasm for life and our interest in the way we look. When a woman stops admiring her own body and even accepting the way it looks, she allows the aging process to set in.

The mechanism of aging

The mechanism of aging is not completely known. There are several theories. One of them (hormonal theory) proposes that aging results from imbalance between old and new cells. This is caused by two related factors: our hormones "age" and the contact between the hormones and our cells becomes weak. Hormones are the means our brain uses to communicate with our cells.

Each cell has receptors that receive the hormonal signals. When the receptors do not react to hormones anymore, the cell undergoes

141

aging and eventually dies. To use a simplistic analogy, our body is like a TV set, our brain like a remote control able to turn it on or off and switch channels, hormones are like the remote control's batteries and finally the receptors are like the contacts connecting the batteries with the remote control.

When the batteries get old, they still work for a while but cause oxidation on the contacts' surfaces. Even though there is nothing wrong with the TV set or the remote control, the system starts working erratically and eventually quits working at all. If the batteries are replaced and the contacts cleaned, everything starts working again. Something similar takes place in our body but the process is more complicated. This, however, is only one of the theories. Our body works according to a blueprint provided by nature; nevertheless the number of years we live on this planet depends largely on our daily attitude towards our body's maintenance.

The art of staying young

There is now a new generation of artificial hormones that are believed to cause no side effects. They can be put in our body; however, the practice shows that the new hormones are only able to slow down the aging process and in some cases they do not bring the expected results at all. On the other hand, according to scientists, we use only 10% of our brain's potential. This means that we have a large reserve of mental abilities that can be put to work.

Memory is a wonderful gift of nature. Our memories engage emotions and emotions in turn, especially the positive ones, put hormones (such as endorphins - the happiness hormones) to work and along with hormones they put cell receptors to work in our entire body.

This means that our positive thoughts and emotions act as the elixir of youth. Regardless of our age, we can always use such thoughts and emotions to move back the arms of our biological clock.

The recipe for staying young

To make good use of our memory, we can pick the memories of our youth, our first affection, and other most happy times of our life from its stores. For a human being (especially female) there is no greater remedy against disease than love.

In the old days, a woman kept her wedding dress and took it out from time to time to admire or even to put it on. It helps to regularly watch the photos from our youth and reunite with our school friends. All these activities serve as the elixir of youth for our mind and body. **Constant orientation towards youth and health not only delays aging – it can even bring back our youth.**

Ancient wisdom contains many adages about staying young and healthy. I selected the most effective ones hoping that they can serve you well. Use them to extend your youth, enjoy good health, and delay the old age as much as possible. Here they are:

1. Love yourself the way you are.
2. Do not envy anybody.
3. If you do not like yourself, make changes in your life.
4. Anger, insults, and criticism of yourself and others are very harmful to your health.
5. If you make a decision, act on it.
6. Joyfully help the poor, ill, and elderly.
7. Never think about diseases, old age, or death.
8. Love is the best remedy against illness and aging.
9. Gluttony, greed, and inability to overcome your weaknesses are your enemies.
10. Worrying causes you to leave this world.
11. Fear and corruption are the worst sins.
12. The best day of your life is today.
13. The best town is where you feel fortunate.
14. The best occupation is the one you enjoy.
15. Losing hope is the worst mistake.
16. The greatest gift you can give or receive is love.
17. Health is your most valuable possession.

Dear readers, I would like you to carefully read the following thought. Properly understood, it can change your life:

To live long and be healthy, we have to be more joyful in our daily life. It is not a skill that anybody can teach us. We have to learn it on our own.

The secrets of wrinkles

Most people look less frequently in the mirror, as they get older. It is hard to come to terms with the fact that our eyes, once large and beautiful, are now partially covered with swollen eyelids hanging over them and conspicuous rounded bags under the eyes make our face look old and unhappy.

We do not want to age and watch new wrinkles showing up on our body and face with resentment. Not many of us fully realize that the image in the mirror is a reflection of our lifestyle. No matter how much we try to cover up our aging with expensive creams and other modern cosmetics, the real condition of our body still becomes apparent. Wrinkles, skin spots, the brightness of our eyes and the shine of our hair, the condition of our nails, and the way we walk or even write reflect the condition of our internal organs. For example, people with an ulcerated stomach or duodenum hunch their back, look pale on their face, and have brown shading under the eyes – typical symptoms of anemia. Another sign of ulceration process in the digestive tract is a white-looking tip of the nose. A deep vertical wrinkle between eyebrows can be connected with frequent strong headaches and the body's demand for more fresh air.

Everything that is happening inside our body manifests itself clearly on the outside. Bags under the eyes can be attributed to something other than aging.

Poorly working kidneys, bladder, or heart causes the bags under the eyes. Similarly, the bags overhanging our eyelids are not a result of sleepless nights as many people believe – they are obvious signs of circulatory system disorders. People have always tried to recognize the condition of internal organs (invisible to the eyes) by watching external signs. The Chinese were first to learn diagnosing diseases based on facial wrinkles. The masters of Sian Min passed their knowledge only to few selected people. Perhaps if many people possessed this knowledge, the general level of health would be much better.

Our appearance – The reflection of our health

This segment will help you understand what our tongue, eyes, lips, hair, skin, etc. can tell us about hidden processes happening inside our

144

body. Even though our body is an integral system where everything is interconnected, it is going to be more convenient here to consider particular parts and how their appearance shows predisposition to certain diseases.

The shape of your head

In many cases, the shape of the head is an indicator of vitality. People with a flat occiput (back of the head) should take into account the possibility that their health may not be very strong by nature. They should try to build up their health using a variety of healing methods. Their most common problems are: constant feeling of weakness, circulatory disorders, migraine headaches, liver pains and digestive tract pains.

Hair

Our hair often determines the way we feel. When our hair becomes unmanageable, hard to style, greasy, dry, or breakable, it is a sign of something wrong going on inside our body. Hair problems are usually caused by inefficient filtering function of the liver or a deficiency in macro- and microelements.

I would like to say a few words to those who are balding. I described in detail the causes of balding and methods of preventing hair loss in my book, "Cure Incurable" (part 1). The letters I received in response to that book indicate that not everybody is able to use those methods in their struggle with hair loss – they asked me for something simpler and easier. I have to disappoint them – there is no easy way. Trying to stop the balding process is a real battle. If you cannot afford the necessary time and energy, change your attitude and do not worry about your balding – there are millions of people like you all over the world. Bald with dignity – do not feel embarrassed and do not try to cover your baldness with the last remaining streak of hair that you grow long for this very purpose. The less attention you pay to your balding the less attention it will draw from other people. There is another comforting fact – French sociologists found that many women associate baldness in men with a pleasant and friendly personality. Don't let your balding bother you too much. After all, what really matters is inside your head.

Forehead

What matters most in the appearance of our forehead is the wrinkles. A cross-shaped wrinkle directly above the base of the nose may indicate a serious spine disorder. Other wrinkles on the forehead signal a tendency to migraine pains caused by degenerated cervical vertebrae. People with broken wavy wrinkles have a poorly balanced nervous system causing them to be short-tempered, prone to depression and despair. A cross-pattern of deep and solid wrinkles indicates a strong personality and resistance to diseases.

Eyes

Our eyes are not only a reflection of our physical health; they also indicate certain traits of our character. They show our vitality as well as wisdom and intelligence.

> *Green eyes* indicate a sensitive and vulnerable personality. People with green eyes are highly dependable. They always crave for Iove and return love with unconditional dedication.
> *Blue eyes* do not suggest a daydreamer or a naive person. To the contrary – blue-eyed people have a strong will, clear goals, and persistency in achieving these goals.
> *Black eyes* mean an erotic nature. Nothing can stand in the way of their desire, especially in romantic matters.
> *Grey eyes* signify an inquiring mind. Gray-eyed people tend to do well in all areas of life, especially in personal relations.
> *Light brown eyes* indicate a reasonable and pragmatic individual.
> *Dark brown eyes* suggest a sensitive temperament, not being clear about life's goals or the means to achieve goals. This often results in moodiness and short temper.

As we know, bags under the eyes result from disorders of our bladder, kidneys, and heart. If we put our efforts towards cleansing these organs, we will remove the cause for the bags and, with time, the bags will disappear. It, hovever, takes some time. If you would like to get rid of the bags sooner, try using the following methods:

Useful advise:

- Pour half a cup of boiling water over a tenspoon of sage, let it stand for 15 minutes, and strain it. Divide the liquid in half; put one half in the refrigerator and leave the other half warm. Soak two cotton pads in the warm brew, lie down comfortably, and put the pads on your lower eyelids for 10 minutes. Next, do the same using pads soaked in the cold brew. Use the routine twice before going to bed every other day for a month. Then make a one-month interval and repeat the therapy.
- Put some chopped up parsley on your lower eyelids and cover with pads soaked in water. Keep it on for 10 minutes before going to bed at least 15 times a month.
- Grate half a potato; blend with an equal amount of wheat flour and cooled down boiled milk. Put the mixture over your eyelids for 15 minutes, then rinse it off with warm water (best mineral water), and put on a conditioning cremn.

Kyebrows can be an indicator of the body's hormonal system.

Eyelids can show stress put on the nervous system. Large eyelids mean normal functioning of the system. A wrinkle along the eyelid means an imbalance of minerals, sleep deprivation, or excessive strain put on the body.

The nose can give clues about qualities of the mind. People with noses bent to the right tend to enjoy physical work; a nose bent to the left suggests interests of intellectual nature.

Lips – The upper lip's shape and color indicate the composition of blood. Lower lip's appearance suggests the condition of internal organs in the lower part of the body.

Teeth – Healthy teeth resemble ivory in color (do not confuse with yellowish smokers' teeth). Overall health of the body is reflected in an attractive shape and uniform color of the teeth. Bad teeth mean poor health. The main cause of teeth decay in our times is consuming cooked and fried foods, products with high sugar content, ice cream, artificial foods, coffee, and sweet beverages.

Improper diet from early childhood leads to a complete deterioration of calcium processing in our body, what is eventually reflected in the condition of our bones and teeth.

Teeth need proper nutrition and cleaning to be healthy. Food should be chewed slowly. Hot or cold food is to be avoided. There should be regular dental check-ups (every six months).

The tongue is the mirror of our body. Based on the tongue's appearance, it can be accurately determined whether the person is in good health. The condition of the tongue can tell us, that a disease is not totally cured even when other symptoms are gone. Diseases of the digestive organs (stomach, liver, intestines) manifest themselves very clearly on the tongue's surface. Most people have a grayish-white lining on their tongue – a sign of digestive disorders. Improper diet leads to acidity of the blood, which promotes the development of disease-causing parasites (yeast, other fungi, etc.) Acidity of the blood is the cause of many disorders the digestive tract, heart, liver, and nervous system. A grayish-white fungal lining on the tongue means an urgent need to change the lifestyle, cleanse the entire body, start combining foods properly, and eat more foods increasing our blood's alkalinity (fruits and vegetables, freshly squeezed juices).

Our ears reflect our creative abilities. People with large ears tend to strive for perfection and knowledge. Small ears mean light-mindedness, limited abilities, and being prone to fatigue.

The chin indicates the strength of character. A chin shifted back means a weak will, low endurance, and proneness to neurasthenia.

The neck shows the biological age. A short neck suggests tendency to circulatory disorders and predisposition to strokes. Short-necked people should keep their body weight down, watch their cholesterol level, and spend more time outdoors.

Long-necked people have a predisposition for angina, bronchitis, and pneumonia. They should increase their immunity against weather changes, breathe through the nose, and prevent colds.

Shoulders

- The left shoulder sitting higher than the right means a predisposition to rheumatism.

148

- Pains in the right shoulder blade indicate disorders of the liver and gallbladder.
- Pain in the left shoulder blade is a sign of stomach ulceration.
- Both shoulders raised suggest a disorder in the functioning of the lungs.
- Both shoulders shifted forward indicate low lung capacity or misalignment of the first spinal segment.
- Both shoulders shifted back signal respiratory disorders (possible asthma).

The skin is the most important breathing organ. For good health, we should get our skin in contact with air and water as much as possible and also (within reason) expose it to sunlight.

Even though all changes on our skin reflect the condition of our internal organs, we can still use natural cosmetics to improve its looks. Potatoes, for example, can be very useful.

Useful advice:

If your skin is dry and discolored, try rubbing it with a blend of two tablespoons of freshly squeezed potato juice and a teaspoon of milk.

To remove discolorations and freckles from a greasy skin, rub a blend of one tablespoon of freshly squeezed potato juice and five drops of lemon juice on it.

Those with visibly expanded capillary vessels can try the following mask: Cut out openings for your eyes, mouth, and nose in a piece of cotton cloth. Soak the cloth in potato juice and put on your face for 30 minutes.

If you have redness on your face as a result of high secretion in the stomach, drink a glass of freshly squeezed potato juice three times a day after meals.

People more advanced in years can use a mask from a cooked potato – cook a potato with the peel, crush it and, while it is still warm, put it on your face. If the skin is withered and dry, add an egg yolk to the potato. Keep the mask on for 30 minutes. Then wipe your face with a milk-soaked piece of cloth if you have a dry skin. For oily skin, use a cloth soaked in warm boiled water. After that, put a lotion on your face and take a look in the mirror – you are going to look younger.

Part Five

SOME FOOD
FOR THOUGHT

Questions and answers

I have had two heart attacks. I used to be obese. In the last two years I managed to reduce my weight by 22lb (10 kg). I would like to stay alive, physically fit, and see my wonderful beloved grandchildren grow up. Professor, give me some advice to maintain a reasonably healthy heart. **Beata B. (61 years old)**

Before I answer your specific question, I would like to make a few general remarks to all my readers.

There is much talk about life "in the fast lane" causing heart attacks. We use terms such as "stress" or "daily tensions" to explain higher mortality rates due to heart attacks. I would not make the connection between nervous tension and heart attacks, particularly among younger population. The cause is simpler: The body is poisoned internally as a result of an improper lifestyle. Insoluble calcium salts and deposits of bad cholesterol damage blood vessels. In addition, blood is thick and acidic, which inevitably causes clots in the blood vessels. This means that all people who do not start taking care of their heart early enough can, sooner or later, expect a heart attack.

I have known many people who did not discriminate in their food and drink choices, did not put any limits on the amounts they consumed, and could spend entire nights in front of computer screens in offices filled with tobacco smoke and strong coffee aroma. They never had time for a walk and their phone was ringing almost 24 hours a day. They often believed to be in good shape because they were not suffering from any pains. Even when they fell down with a heart attack, they still refused to blame their lifestyle for it. According to them, the cause was the work-related stress and daily worries. As we know from history, human beings have always lived under stress. We cannot even imagine the stress our distant ancestors must have experienced when they were in danger of being attacked by a wild animal at any moment. They had very limited means of protecting themselves against cataclysms such as hurricanes, earthquakes, or floods and sheltering from elements such as wind, sun, rain, or snow. Our genes preserved the ability to resist stress – life has always been full of stress, there is nothing new about it. To live means to contend with stress coming from all directions 24 hours a day.

Some readers may argue that our ancestors usually died before the age of forty. It is true - we live longer now. But do we live better? People are often physically fit until the age of 40-50 and then suffer a heart attack or stroke. They live partially disabled for another 20 years, cannot fully enjoy their life, and have to worry about being a burden to their families.

Many people who are busy making money for 15-20 years and destroy their health in the process reflect sadly that they are ready to give the money away in return for the lost health. Had they thought about it earlier, they would have been able to enjoy both health and prosperity. I feel sincerely sorry for those who spend years building a career but are not willing to spend even five minutes taking care of their health.

All businessmen and businesswomen would probably argue that it is easy for me to give such advice from a country retreat or a quiet office, while they have to contend with daily stress and worries, can afford only three to five hours of sleep, and hardly have time to swallow a pill when something goes wrong with their health.

In reply I would inform them that I think about the content of my future books while I take morning power walks (6-7.5 miles / 10-12km) that allow me to maintain a good shape, a strong heart, and excellent memory. I have had difficult times in my life when I was not able to walk, not even get out of bed for two years because of spinal injury. However, my love for life and the desire to be healthy allowed me to heal my spine and start helping others in dealing with similar problems.

Your strong determination is a very positive factor that will help you stay alive and healthy. In my life, I have met many people that were physically fit, or even had athletic achievements, despite their history of heart attacks. An acquaintance of mine ran in15.6-mile (about 25km) marathons at the age of sixty – ten years after his heart attack.

The cells of our body have a miraculous ability to regenerate themselves. Our heart muscle can be rebuilt and made strong, just like all other muscles. It is not an easy task after a heart attack, but it is possible.

When we think about heart disease, we should look at the entire circulatory system – including all vessels and veins that carry our blood. The condition of our blood vessels is the reflection of our heart's functioning, its endurance, and reliability. Our biological age is determined not by the number of years but, in a large degree, the state of the capillary vessels and veins, their flexibility, cleanliness, and the ability to react to all kinds of stresses (nervous tension, noise, temperature and humidity changes, etc.).

If you are looking for a complete program designed to maintain a healthy heart, read the sections about exercise, breathing, water therapies, and body cleansing. Even though they are not about heart disease as such, advice contained there helps improve the health of the entire body including the heart, one of our body's most vital organs.

In short, the health of our heart depends on the good condition of the rest of our circulatory system, e.g. the quality of our blood (its alkalinity) and the efficient functioning of our liver and kidneys. The way to achieve this is:

1. An active lifestyle.
2. A diet consisting mainly of plant-based food products.
3. Regularly cleansing your body of the toxic products of metabolism by using the therapies presented in this book for body cleansing and strengthening the circulatory system (e.g. garlic extract, page 91, lemon therapy, page 90, or recipes in the chapter "Health without medications"). This needs to be done even if you maintain a very hygienic lifestyle.
4. Realizing that the process of regeneration (rebuilding) of our blood vessels and heart has to be gradual. We often start causing damage to our circulatory system from 8-10 years of age (a hidden form of arteriosclerosis). To reverse the damage done over a number of years, we have to proceed in small, reasonable steps.

A good comprehension of the overall philosophy of healthy lifestyle contained in this book would allow you to stop your heart problems once and for all.

I do not believe that a proper diet can allow me to live up to 150 years. **Jacek K.**

You are probably still young and do not worry much about your health. The older we get the more we understand and appreciate the gift of good health. We want not only to live longer but also to avoid disease. Correct diet is sure to extend our life and, what is even more important, enjoy good health.

We can rely on the longevity record of Hunza Valley inhabitants in India. The average longevity among 32,000 inhabitants is 120 years. What is their secret?

Scottish physician McCarrison who lived 15 years in the area of Hunza Valley concluded that the main reason for the inhabitants' longevity is their diet. They are vegetarians and their usual diet consists of raw fruits and vegetables in the summer; in the winter it consists mainly of grain sprouts, dried apricots, and sheep cheese.

On his return to England McCarrison conducted a series of experiments with animals, in order to be finally convinced about the connection between diet and longevity. One group of animals was fed the diet of a typical London family (white bread, herrings, refined sugar, canned and cooked vegetables, etc. It resulted in various "human" disorders among the animals. The other group of animals, fed a "Hunza Valley diet", remained healthy throughout the experiments.

It is believed that climate influences longevity. It is an interesting fact that other groups of people living in similar climates to that of Hunza Valley suffer from many health disorders and their longevity is two times shorter. The mountain climate does not prevent them from diseases because their diet is not healthy.

Hunza Valley inhabitants, in contrast to neighboring ethnic groups, look very much like Europeans. Historians propose a theory that merchants and soldiers who settled in Hunza Valley during the expedition of Alexander the Great along the Indus River started the tribal communities there. That means even Europeans can live long if they eat properly.

What would you say about the consumption of alcohol? People continue to drink even though there is so much information about its harmfulness. Is alcohol harmful or not?
Krzysztof K.

There is a very wise ancient saying: There are three things that are very harmful when used excessively and very beneficial in moderate amounts – bread, salt, and wine. I wrote earlier about bread and salt. Let's take a look at wine.

Since our childhood, we hear much about the harmful effects of alcohol consumption – I would not be able to say anything new about that. I suggest we also consider some health benefits of moderate alcohol consumption.

Once I have seen an interesting cartoon. Animals in the Kalahari Desert gathered to have a meal together. Berries used for the meal were partially fermented. As an effect of eating the berries, the animals became very peaceful – predators and prey, lions and antelopes, tigers and elephants were all very happy and forgot about hatred and aggression. It turns out that mammals (including humans, the most developed ones) need small amounts of alcohol. It causes our brain to release "the hormone of happiness", relaxing the muscles, lowering our concentration and the tension of our nervous system. We receive all these benefits only if we use alcohol in small amounts, treating it like a medication. Hippocrates also believed that alcohol in moderate amounts is appropriate for both the healthy and the ill.

In the opinion of Louis Pasteur, wine has the full right to be considered the healthiest of all beverages if used with moderation. Ancient Greek philosophers often repeated to their followers: "The power of gods can hardly equal the usefulness of wine," and the old Eastern adage says: "Everybody can drink as long as they know the right time, place, amount, and can afford it."

This kind of reasoning can be found in the opinions of many respected thinkers. Our troubles begin when we forget about moderation. This applies to all aspects of life, not only to eating and drinking.

Determining what we mean by "moderate amount" is more complicated – it can have different meanings for different people. American researchers, based on many years of studies, suggest the following amounts as harmless: 1g of wine or 0.25g of liquor per 1kg of body weight a day. Different kinds of wine influence our health differently. For example, **white wine** cleanses the kidneys, slightly stimulates the nervous system, and improves digestion. **Red wine** improves the functioning of our liver, calms the nervous system, improves breathing processes, and lowers the risk of heart disease in people with high cholesterol level.

The information presented below can be useful for anybody – from abstainers to heavy drinkers. Studies conducted in different coun-

157

tries reached some common conclusions about the influence of drinking wine on different systems in our body:

1. It positively affects the nervous system and stimulates the endocrine glands.
2. It improves digestion (of animal protein in particular) by stimulating the secretion of gastric juices.
3. It helps maintain the proper pH level of the gastric juices.
4. By positively influencing the digestive system, it slightly relieves the stress on the entire body.
5. Liver cells stimulated by alcohol supply more bile to the duodenum.
6. Potassium salts present in wine and brandy have a diuretic effect on the kidneys.
7. Stimulated breathing centers improve the ventilation of the lungs.
8. It improves the cardiovascular system by causing the vessels to expand and contract, which has a massaging effect.
9. Alcohol flushes toxic products (e.g. phenol) out of the body.
10. The delicate aroma stimulates our smell centers.
11. Alcohol has disinfecting and antitoxic qualities.
12. It prevents the accumulation of fat on the walls of blood vessels, reducing the risk of cardiovascular disorders.

There have been many studies in recent years concerning the influence of alcohol on the heart muscle. Some American researchers concluded that every beverage containing alcohol strengthens the heart. They particularly point out the high content of natural antioxidants in red wine. It was noticed that people who never consume any alcoholic beverages suffer much more frequently from heart disorders. English and Swiss scientists concluded that alcohol in moderate amounts reduces the risk of heart attacks by 40% and the disorders of blood vessels by 20%.

I would like to stress that wine drinking is particularly beneficial for the elderly and for people suffering from anemia or weak health in general.

There is a saying in Burgundy: "Wine is the milk for the elderly." It is advisable for people over fifty to prepare and consume the "longevity drink" once a week (best on Sunday with a group of good friends). It is especially helpful for women going through menopause.

"Longevity drink" preparation: In a pot, mix two bottles of sweet or semi-sweet wine with 0.5 liter of water. Boil it for 10 minutes using low heat; add a pinch of clove buds, cinnamon, and cardamom, and 10 slices of peeled lemon and then boil for another 5 minutes. Finally add one tablespoon of brandy, turn off the heat, cover the pot with a lid, and let it stand for 20 minutes. Strain the mixture and drink while it is still warm (this recipe is for 10 servings – divide the amounts by 10 if you want to prepare just one serving).

I am sixty years old and have been trying to fight osteoporosis for the last 10 years. It is a lost battle so far. Do you know any remedies? **Malgorzata F.**

In my book "Cure incurable", part one, pages 11-31, I described the therapies to be used against this debilitating disease in detail. I was glad to receive many letters from the readers confirming amazingly good positive effects of therapies suggested in the book.

This is more proof that there are no incurable diseases. I always stress that patience and knowledge about our own body can overcome any disease. I will give some useful advice for you and others who suffer form osteoporosis, but I have to start with some explanations.

Two forms of calcium

There are two forms of calcium in our food products. Good, organic calcium that is easily absorbed into our bones is found in vegetables, fruits (especially the peel), freshly squeezed juices, eggs, bran, wheat and oat sprouts, nuts, honey, and fresh cow or goat milk. Bad, non-organic, hard to absorb form of calcium is contained in all refined products, bread, pasteurized or cooked milk and their products, boiled water; all products processed in temperatures over 212F/100C (cooked, fried, etc.), and synthetically produced calcium formulas. If our diet consists mainly of refined food products, pasteurized or boiled milk, crunchy bread, cooked or fried products, and if the water we use is usually boiled (this is true for most people), it is obvious why our bones are so often affected by osteoporosis.

The causes of calcium deficiency

Among the different elements in our body, the amount of calcium is the fifth after the four basic elements: carbon, oxygen, hydrogen, and nitrogen. On the average, there is about 2.6lb (1.2kg) of calcium in a human body and 99% of this amount is contained in the bones.

Besides supporting our body (keeping in the vertical position), the bone tissue has the function of storing calcium and phosphorus, so that the body can have an emergency supply of these elements when it does not get an adequate amount from the food we eat. The level of calcium in blood is at a constant level – even in the last stages of osteoporosis the blood can maintain 99.9% of the required level by taking calcium from the bones. If our blood has to take calcium from the bones day after day, the bone mass starts diminishing.

It is known that products such as meat, cheese, sugar, and animal fats produce large amounts of harmful acids (lactic, oxalic, uric, and other) when they are digested. Calcium salts are used to neutralize these acids and protect our body from poisoning. The more of these products we eat the less calcium is left in our bones.

One of the main causes of calcium deficiency is high consumption of sugar and products containing sugar. It is a synthetic product and its digestion results in many poisonous acids in our body. Huge amounts of mineral salts containing mostly calcium are needed to neutralize these acids. Where are they taken from? They are taken from our bones and teeth, where they are present in the highest concentration. Considering the fact that we develop a taste for sweets from early childhood and even adults consume every day hundreds of times more sugar than the safe amount, it is obvious why children suffer from tooth decay, adults from gum disease, and the bones of the elderly are as porous as Swiss cheese (osteoporosis).

In conclusion, one of the main causes of osteoporosis is excessive liking for sweets passed down from generation to generation. I often hear parents say: "How can I refuse my child a candy. Childhood should be sweet." I would advise parents to think more about providing a healthy and happy childhood for their offspring. When the children grow old, pleasures of their sweet childhood may cost them years of suffering from bone and spine pains.

Another cause of osteoporosis is lack of physical exercise. I have covered the topic of exercise before. I can only add here that the less time we spend being physically active the higher our risk of becoming ill with osteoporosis.

The most likely factors contributing to the risk of osteoporosis, based on the observation of patients, (including those who got cured) are the following:

1. Deficiency in vitamins D and C
2. Diet rich in thermally processed products
3. Using mainly boiled water
4. Not enough fruits, vegetables, and their freshly squeezed juices in the diet
5. Eating fruits and vegetables without peel
6. Improperly prepared meals (long cooking and frying)
7. Overeating
8. Smoking
9. Lack of exercise
10. High consumption of milk
11. High consumption of bread and other flour-based products
12. High consumption of sugar and sweets
13. High consumption of animal fats
14. Taking large amounts of synthetic vitamins
15. Eating refined products containing insoluble (non-organic) calcium: pre-cooked grains, pasta, ready-made soups and other

If you honestly considered all of the above points, you would probably have to put a checkmark next to each of them. This would mean you are sure to become ill with osteoporosis or you are ill already without knowing about it.

What you have to do now is to eliminate all these factors from your lifestyle. If you already need a therapy, the most effective ones are:

1. Lemon therapy
2. Eggshell therapy

Lemon therapy

Use only pure lemon juice for the purpose of this therapy – do not dilute it with water; do not add any honey or sugar. It should be prepared the same way as for preventative lemon therapy (Page 90). You can drink it half an hour before or one hour after your meals, which-ever is more convenient. To treat serious, chronic diseases, we have to drink in total juice squeezed from 200 lemons during the therapy. This number might surprise you. Some people get a sensation of sour taste in their mouth just by thinking about such amount of citric acid. This is not an error – it has to be 200 lemons and not even one fewer (more is allowed).

During my practice, I have seen hundreds of people who enjoyed good health thanks to drinking large amounts of lemon juice. I drank up to ten cups of lemon juice (squeezed from about forty lemons) daily. When you try, you will find out that there is nothing to be afraid of. In rare cases, large amounts of citric acid in the stomach may lead to irregularities of intestinal function. In such cases we can temporarily switch to preventative therapy dosages until our stomach gets used to lemon juice, and then try the healing therapy again.

In healing therapy, the following dosages are recommended:

> Day 1 & 12 – 5 lemons
> Day 2 & 11 – 10 lemons
> Day 3 & 10 – 15 lemons
> Day 4 & 9 – 20 lemons
> Day 5,6,7 and 8 – 25 lemons

This represents in total juice squeezed from 200 lemons consumed over 12 days. The daily amounts should be split into 3-5 dosages. Some people are terrified by the amount of juice (about one liter or quart) to be consumed on days 5, 6, 7, and 8. However, we are not afraid to drink two quarts of apple or blackcurrant juice. Lemon is just another fruit only more sour.

The therapy described above can be used for treating kidney stones. Lemon juice is one of the best remedies against them. There is an observable increase in the kidney function during the therapy. Your urine may get darker and, when allowed to stand for some time, may produce reddish sediment of uric salts. At the beginning of the therapy, one quart of urine can produce a significant amount of sediment. This means that uric acid is rapidly removed from our body thanks to the therapy. Our urine becomes amber-colored at the end of the therapy and it does not produce sediment even if allowed to stand for a long time. This means that our body does not contain excess amounts of uric acid anymore.

Lemon juice therapy is the best way to replenish vitamins in our body. We chronically suffer from vitamin deficiency, especially those who smoke (one cigarette destroys up to 25mg of vitamin C, which is a quarter of our daily recommended intake). There are still many smokers among us. Lemon juice offers wonderful benefits because citric acid is the only acid that reacts with calcium in our body, forming unique salt. As this salt is dissolved, our body receives calcium and phosphorus - elements that normalize metabolism and regenerate bone tissue.

Citric acid is also one of the products of our complex digestive process. If we supply it in the form of lemon juice, besides reducing thirst we allow our body to save energy, which can then be used for removing salty deposits from our bones, joints, muscles, and blood vessels. When citric acid reacts with amines, it forms aspartic acid that has negative charge. Natural aspartic acid formed in our body during lemon juice therapy is very valuable. Practically all pharmaceutical formulas used in treating diseases, which were described above, contain aspartic acid in its synthetic form.

Here is some more advice on the usefulness of lemon. In cases of sore throat or early symptoms of sore throat, suck on a slice of lemon every 15 minutes - even small amounts of diluted citric acid are able to kill all germs. If you suffer from gum disease or sore gums, rinse your mouth regularly with a solution of lemon juice and warm boiled water in the morning and the evening for two weeks.

Lemon is also very effective for strengthening hair. If you have dandruff and weak hair, rub the skin on your head with a slice of lemon once a day for ten days. This will strengthen your hair and stop the formation of dandruff. Boldness is described in my book "Cure incurable", part one.

Eggshell therapy

Eggshells are not trash. They are helpful in the treatment of osteoporosis. They are an ideal source of calcium that is 90% absorbable by our bones. Besides calcium carbonate, eggshells contain all the microelements essential for our body: copper, fluorine, iron, manganese, molybdenum, sulfur, silicon, zinc, and other - 27 elements in total. The

163

composition of an eggshell is very similar to that of our bones and teeth. German and Hungarian scientists who researched the influence of eggshell therapy on the human body concluded that for both children and adults it had positive results against breaking nails and hair, bleeding gums, constipation, hypersensitivity, insomnia, chronic colds, and asthma. The therapy strengthens the bone tissue and removes radioactive elements from the body.

Eggshell therapy offers invaluable benefits in the treatment and prevention of osteoporosis without causing any side effects. The therapy is simple and does not require any expenses.

Recipe

Immerse an eggshell in boiling water for 5 minutes, let it dry, and grind it in a coffee grinder. Take 0.01-0.02oz (0.5-1g) a day. You can mix it with juice squeezed from one half of a lemon or add it to your grains and cottage cheese for osteoporosis prevention. Use this therapy for 30 days twice a year (January and November).

Black radish leave recipe

Juice from black radish leaves is a very effective remedy for children and adults against the abnormal softening of tooth and bone tissue (osteomalacia). For best effects, use a blend of juices squeezed from black radish leaves (3.2oz/90g), dandelions (3.2oz/90g), and carrots (9.9oz/280g) for two servings - in the morning and the evening.

Let us sum up all steps you should undertake if you are ill with osteoporosis:

1. Change your diet - avoid products that flush calcium out of your bones (coffee, animal fats, etc.)
2. Drink freshly squeezed fruit juices (at least two glasses a day).
3. Make sure your diet contains an adequate amount of natural vitamins (particularly vitamin C).
4. Eat one ground eggshell, one soft-boiled egg, and one apple every day.
5. Regularly eat beans, peas, broccoli, and oats - they all are rich in estrogens.
6. Use cleansing therapies presented in this book.

7. Take alternate hot and cold showers in the morning and the evening.
8. Strengthen your bones by daily exercise (for example, dance and jump to the sounds of your favorite music for 10-15 minutes).

I am 21 years old. Since childhood, I have been suffering from large intestine troubles (frequent constipation). I got hemorrhoids at the age of 16, and they got worse after I delivered a baby. The doctors suggest surgical removal. I am afraid and do not want a surgery. Please give me some alternative advice. **Lidia M**.

Surgical removal of hemorrhoids benefits everybody involved except the patient. As a rule, hemorrhoids show up again after some time because the surgery does not remove their causes.

Hemorrhoids (dilated veins in the lower part of the large intestine) usually happen to people who habitually consume large amounts of bread, sweets, coffee, tea, and all kinds of sandwiches with bread and deli products.

Hemorrhoids are, among others, a sign of inefficient circulatory system, inflexible blood vessels and veins, and thickness of blood caused by deficiency in natural minerals found in vegetables and fruits. Contact of your anus with cold surfaces can also be a cause of hemorrhoids. Women often get hemorrhoids after child delivery and resulting dislocation of lumbar vertebrae.

A likely cause of hemorrhoids in men can be a large body mass, especially a conspicuous belly. Another major factor is a sedentary lifestyle leading to constipation and eventually hemorrhoids.

Since we know the causes, we can develop a plan of action:

1. Lead a more active lifestyle. In particular, exercise muscles in the lower part of your body.
2. Limit the consumption of sweets, bread, tea, and coffee. Eat more raw or cooked vegetables and fruits.
3. Prevent constipation by cleansing your large intestine. Build up healthy intestinal microflora (see page 188).

165

4. Learn to eat slowly and do not drink at your meals. This is a fundamental rule for good functioning of your digestive system, especially your large intestine.

Then you can try a few therapies described below.

- Cut a stick (about as thick as your little finger) out of a raw potato and put in your rectum for the night. Use the therapy every other night for two weeks.
- Instead of using toilet paper after stools, wash your anus with alternately warm and cold water (five times each) and dry gently with a soft towel.
- Put 2 tablespoons of tobacco in a plastic bucket that is comfortable to sit on. Pour one quart (about 1L) of boiling water over it, put a lid on, and let it stand for 20 minutes. When the steam is not too hot anymore, take off the lid and sit on top of the bucket for 3-5 minutes.
- Drink the following juice blends 15 minutes before meals:
  - 1.8oz/50g carrot + 1.4oz/40g celery + 0.7oz/20g parsnips + 1.05oz/30g spinach
  - 3.2oz/90g carrot + 2.1oz/60g spinach
- Put an ice cube wrapped in cotton cloth into your rectum for 5-10 seconds. Use this therapy after stools (when you use a wash instead of toilet paper) for 1-2 months.
- To get rid of hemorrhoids for good, switch to strictly fruit-and-vegetable diet for two weeks during summer months. Do not eat any meat, white flour products, or dairy products; do not drink coffee, cocoa, chocolate, or alcoholic beverages. You can eat small amounts of walnuts instead of bread and drink raspberry, currant, mint, or chamomile tea.

Finally, another important remark: **suffering from hemorrhoids brings you a step closer to becoming ill with colon cancer.**

Can you tell me the simplest preventative methods against cancer? **Justyna D.**

I am sorry, but there is no universal method. In one of my radio interviews, I answered this question the following way:

- Eat fruits and vegetables grown in your geographical region and drink their freshly squeezed juices. There should be at least one apple and raw or cooked vegetables in your menu every day. Most valuable are vegetables and fruits with intensive green, orange, or red color (spinach, lettuce, cucumber, beans, peas, tomatoes, beets, carrot, pumpkin, pears, apples, etc.). They supply our body with all essential vitamins, minerals, fiber, and oxygen.
- Know the difference among many kinds of fats. Fats are necessary for our body, especially at an advanced age. What kinds of fats are better? Plant oils, especially cold-pressed ones, contain acids and vitamins that extend our longevity. It is a good idea to take one teaspoon of oil every morning and evening and also to add one tablespoon of oil to your salads. The intake of meat, milk, and margarine should be limited.
- Use more outdoor physical activity and learn to breathe correctly. Oxygen contained in the air is essential for each one of the billions of cells in our body and helps them regenerate, slowing down the aging process. Physical activity allows oxygen to reach all cells – this is why it is better to exercise outdoors.
- Be joyful! Your emotions affect not only your mind – they influence most physiological reactions in your body. When we are worried or irritated, our immune system (our body's natural defense system) stops issuing hormones T and B, which among others protect us from infections and cancer. When we are happy and enjoy our life, our immune system gets stronger and can better protect our health.
- Find time to relax. Life in our modern world is full of tension and stress. They cannot be avoided but they should not be accumulated. Allow yourself time to do what you enjoy – go to your room and listen to favorite music, meditate, or take a walk in the woods. It helps to spend some time alone (3-5 minutes), relax, and forget all your troubles.
- Keep your mind busy. The more your brain works the more stress it is able to bear. Regardless of your age, stimulate brain centers responsible for your memory. Read books, visit museums, listen to lectures, and play chess – in other words, use your head.

- Get adequate amounts of sleep. Restful sleep clears the mind, relaxes muscles, reduces blood pressure, regenerates the hormonal system, and increases immunity. Even wounds heal better during sleep. People who are deprived of sleep for a few days show symptoms of psychological problems. Our demand for sleep varies. For some of us 4-5 hours is adequate while others need 8-10 hours. We should allow ourselves as much sleep as our body demands. This means that we should feel rested and refreshed when we get up.
- Learn to enjoy walking. It is one of the ways to keep your immune system strong. Maintaining the temperature in your bedroom at 61-63F (about16-17C) and taking alternate hot and cold showers every morning and evening also help develop your immunity.
- Eat less; apply the principle of eating to live instead of living to eat. Chew your food slowly and leave the table while you still feel a slight sensation of hunger. Eat more natural products that do not undergo thermal processing (especially long frying).
- Laugh more. Laughter engages more muscles than you realize. It massages our internal organs and stimulates the digestive system. It relieves pain and removes inflammations. We breathe deeper when we laugh, supplying more oxygen to our lungs. Our brain produces serotonin – the "happiness hormone." Finally, laughter often breaks the barriers in relations with other people.
- Make love. Ancient medicine saw aspects of immortality in the union of male and female elements. The erotic act best rebuilds the harmony of our body.
- Cleanse your body. Remember that its internal condition is going to be reflected in your external appearance.
- Tune into what your body is telling you. The body can appreciate your concern. If you want to remain healthy, take care of yourself before the illness strikes.

I cannot get rid of heavy sweating of my palms and feet. Nothing I have tried helps against this problem. I developed phobias because of this and try not to go out because it makes me nervous and increases my sweating. **Jan N.**

First of all, we can learn to control our nervous system by some psychological exercises and stop constantly thinking about our sweating problem. Second, reduce meat in your diet because it is the cause of our sweat's offensive odor. Cleanse your body and get it used to temperature changes (by using alternate showers). Here are some practical ways to get rid of unpleasant foot odor:

1. Take some fresh birch twigs, crush them, put between your toes, put socks on, and wear it for at least 2 hours.
2. Put some powdered oak bark in your socks, put the socks on and keep them on overnight. Wash your feet with warm water in the morning and towel dry. Repeat every other day for two weeks.
3. Put some powdered boric acid in your socks; wear the socks overnight, wash your feet with cold water in the morning, and towel dry. Repeat every other day for two weeks.
4. Keep your feet under a stream of running cold water every morning and evening for 5-10 seconds over the period of 90 days. This simple method is helpful not only against excessive sweating but also against throat diseases and it can be used throughout your entire life.

You wrote in one of your articles that taking synthetic vitamin C is harmful. Why is that? **Maria K.**

It is not only vitamin C – all synthetic vitamins are harmful.

First: Most vitamins are compounds formed by plants in the process of biosynthesis under the influence of sunlight. Vitamins in plants are in forms (provitamins) that are easily absorbed by the human body. Plants also contain all mineral salts and other compounds (some still unknown) that help in full absorption of vitamins. This is why it is impossible to overdose natural vitamins, unlike the synthetic ones.

Second: Artificial vitamins are non-organic crystalloid substances treated as foreign substances by our body. They are absorbed with difficulty or not absorbed at all (especially in case of metabolic disorders). This is why many people notice that their urine has the color and

169

smell of the vitamins. There are frequent cases of rejection in the form of nausea, weakness, or itching.

Third: One of the side effects of taking synthetic vitamins is increased appetite. This happens because the body, in order to absorb the vitamins, needs additional amounts of mineral salts, carbohydrates, and proteins. Unlike plant-based foods, synthetic vitamins do not have these ingredients and the body instinctively looks for more food, which leads to obesity.

The effects of taking synthetic vitamin C

In most people's mind, vitamin C has the opinion of a harmless supplement. However, in recent years physicians started noticing more and more side effects caused by vitamin C overdosing. It is common that people take vitamin C in liberal amounts, sometimes 0.14-0.21oz (4-6g) a day, as a remedy against flu and some viral infections, while the recommended amount is about 100mg a day.

Scientists in many countries agree with the opinion that taking synthetic vitamin C does not increase immunity against colds, and its large doses make the symptoms of some infectious-allergic diseases (especially rheumatism) more severe.

The most dangerous effect of high doses of vitamin C is increased coagulability of blood, leading to blood clots. Another effect can be formation of stones from oxalic acid and uric acid in the kidneys and bladder.

Synthetic vitamin C destroys other vitamins. Patients who get shots of vitamin B2 are advised by physicians to stop taking vitamin C during that time because of this effect.

Large doses of vitamin C interfere with the production of insulin by the pancreas in diabetics and cause an increase of sugar level in their urine and blood. Recent research shows that vitamin C overdosing slows down the transmission of nerve-muscle impulses, causing increased muscle fatigue and lowering the coordination between eyes and muscles.

Vitamin C is not stored in our body. It is a good idea to consult your physician about the effects of synthetic vitamin C. Natural vitamins found in large amounts in fruits and vegetables are most beneficial – it is not possible to overdose them.

A psychic at a fair told me that I should not wear many rings on my fingers. **Halina C.**

The psychic was absolutely right. There are scientific studies making a connection between some women's disorders and jewelry worn on their fingers.

It is known that there are many contact points on the fingers that are connected with internal organs. For example, a ring on the fourth finger causes disorders of nipples, reproductive organs, and endocrine glands. A ring on the middle finger may cause arteriosclerosis or high blood pressure, a ring on the index finger – back pain, calcification of bones, and inflammations of spinal nerve roots (radiculitis). Frequent wearing of jewelry on the little finger leads to duodenum disorders.

My advice: Do not put unnecessary strain on your hands by excessive use of jewelry. Take off even your wedding ring when going to sleep – your hands need to rest completely from time to time. When you have time (e.g. while watching TV), massage the fingers of your right and left hand in turn, one minute each – massaging our finger influences our eyes. If you do such a massage every day, you will not need glasses and your hands will always feel rested.

Can diet influence the gender of our future child? **Elzbieta and Maciej P.**

There is much evidence accumulated in recent years for the connection between certain products in the parents' diet and the gender of their future child.

On one of the Japanese islands, four times as many boys as girls have been born over many years. Japanese scientists believe that it is caused by drinking local water that has high alkaline content. According to some French researchers, diet determines the gender of a future child in 80% - high potassium content promotes the conception of a boy; high calcium content gives better odds for the conception of a girl.

Products increasing the odds of conceiving a boy: alkaline mineral water, fruit juices, deli products, egg white, potatoes, mushrooms, pea, bananas, dates, apricots, oranges, cherries, dried plums.

Products increasing the odds of conceiving a girl: mineral water rich in calcium, chocolate, cocoa, eggs, cottage cheese, kefir, cream, aged cheese, yeast-free baked goods, eggplant, beets, carrots, cucumbers, onion, peppers, apples, strawberries, raspberries, grapefruits, nuts, sugar, honey, jams.

> *I have been treating prostate gland inflammation without results for many years. Do you know any remedies?*
> **Roman B.**

According to statistics, two out of three males over the age of 45 suffer from this disorder so it is useful to know some facts about it. To detect prostate inflammation in its first stage, we ought to pay attention to the following symptoms:

1. More frequent need to urinate
2. Weak and interrupted urinary flow
3. Interrupted sleep; the need to urinate at night
4. Inability to completely empty the bladder

If these symptoms are ignored and remain untreated, they may result in urinary tract infections, serious kidney disorders, and lower sexual drive. Men over 40 should visit a urologist for a check-up once a year; for those over 55, two visits a year are recommended.

Useful advice:

Preventative steps to be undertaken over the age of 40:

- Avoid a sedentary lifestyle.
- Prevent constipation.
- Prevent your body (especially feet) from getting cold – use warm underwear and do not spend much time in cold temperatures.
- Do not overuse alcohol.
- Try to consume more vegetables, fruits, plain yogurt, kefir, cottage cheese, grains, beets, cabbage, whole grain breads; drink vegetable cocktails from freshly squeezed beet, carrot, and cucumber juice (1:3:1).

- Walk more regardless of the weather.
- Prevent obesity.
- Definitely limit your intake of sugar, its products, and refined flour products.
- Lead an active life, exercise in the morning, and build up immunity to temperature changes (alternate hot and cold showers), especially for your feet (putting under cold water for a short time, massages, walking barefoot on grass, a beach etc.).
- Regular short fasts bring good results (water only 24-36 hours once a week).

I would also like to give some advice for those who already suffer from the disorder.

Genital-urinary tract cleansing:

Put 2 tablespoons of unrefined rice in a half-liter jar, fill the jar with cold boiled water and let it stand for 24 hours. On the second day, add a second jar with rice and water, rinse the rice in the first jar, and change its water. Repeat this for five days adding one more jar every day and changing water in the other jars – you will have five jars with soaked rice. On the sixth day, cook the rice from the first jar for 15 minutes and eat it right away without anything else (you can add some butter or vegetable oil, but no salt). Do not eat or drink anything for the next three hours. Put the empty first jar at the end of the queue as jar #6, put rice in it and fill with water. On the next day, cook and eat rice from jar #2, then use the jar at the end of the queue. Use this routine for two months, eating rice from the oldest jar every day, changing water in all jars, and adding one jar.

The therapy cures prostate inflammations (males) and genital-urinary system inflammations (females).

You write that coffee is harmful. I have read in other sources that drinking coffee has many benefits. **Bozena T.**

If you want to stay healthy, you need to control the amount of coffee you drink. Coffee does not have any nutritional value. It suppresses

173

the absorption of proteins and reduces the levels of necessary micro-elements (iron, calcium) and group B vitamins. Coffee puts a lot of stress on the liver – excessive users feel chills over their body 10-15 minutes after having another cup. French research shows that people who drink over 3 cups a day suffer from a hidden form of anemia. Those whose average daily intake is about six cups show some symptoms of paranoia. In addition, coffee has the ability to retain radionuclides in our body.

American studies conducted over 25 years, and involving 85,000 hospital employees is more optimistic about the issue but it also proves very strong influence of caffeine on the human body.

In conclusion, drinking coffee in moderate amounts has its benefits in the form of antistatic qualities. There are no products totally harmful or totally beneficial – a substance can be a poison or a medicine, depending on the amount. I can only repeat the well-known truth that all depends on moderation. One or two cups of coffee a day should be enough.

Finally, I would like to tell you about interesting research about the effectiveness of commonly used beverages in flushing stones out of our kidneys (on a scale of 0-100%).

1. Coca-Cola: 2%
2. Boiled water: 2-4%
3. Table water: 6-8%
4. Mineral water: 12-18%
5. Black tea: 12%
6. Coffee: 16%
7. Beer: 20%
8. Green tea: 46-60%

There are benefits from drinking mineral water, black tea, coffee, or even beer from time to time, but the most beneficial beverage to be used regularly is green tea.

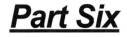

Part Six

COMPLETE BODY CLEANSING

Complete body cleansing consists of external and internal hygiene. The following section of the book deals with the ways of maintaining complete hygiene in order to improve our overall health.

Harmful materials accumulated in our body over many years are the real cause of many diseases. To allow the removal of our body's toxic waste, we first need to unplug all our internal cleaning systems. Complete body cleansing is absolutely necessary if we want to have a harmoniously functioning body that is free of internal contamination. Each stage of the cleansing procedure will bring us observable results. The cleansing of our large intestine will stop bloating, constipation, and heartburn; clean liver brings us better digestion, improved memory, healthy-looking eyes, shiny hair, younger looks, more energy, strength, and endurance. After the cleansing of our kidneys the bags under the eyes disappear, blood pressure stabilizes, and abdominal pains stop; clean joints (free of salty deposits) have a wider range of motion, better flexibility, and do not react to weather changes. Clean lymph and blood vessels prevent us from infections, heart attacks, strokes, varicose veins, and many other disorders.

We like the look of our home after renovations. A clean garment feels good; our car with a brand new paint job is pleasant to the eye. However, none of these feelings come close to the way we feel when our body is completely cleansed. If you decide to take this step, you will feel as if you received a brand new body.

EXTERNAL HYGIENE

Cleaning the teeth

We undoubtedly know more about external body hygiene than about internal hygiene, but this knowledge does not always produce expected effects. Regular teeth brushing, for some people 2-3 times a day is a well-established habit. We brush thoroughly and use good quality toothpastes but many of us still have to deal with tooth decay and gum disease. What is the reason for this?

First, the toothbrushes we use damage our teeth as they clean them. Hard toothbrushes hurt our gums. Particles of food get into the cuts where they start rotting and cause bacterial infections. Second, toothbrushes do not improve blood circulation in the gum because they do not provide good gum massage. Third, toothbrushes themselves are eventually infected with bacteria. For these reasons, even regular and thorough brushing does not prevent people from two disorders: tooth decay (caused by chemical processes on the tooth surface) and periodontal disease (bacterial infection below the gum line, causing damage to the tissue and bone supporting the teeth). These disorders cause not only toothaches but also many other disorders such as joint inflammations; high blood pressure; disorders of kidneys, heart, and stomach; poor functioning of the eyes, nose, and ears. What can we do to avoid all these troubles? We can follow the example of yoga gurus, who originated body-cleansing techniques. They consider the use of regular toothbrushes poor hygiene. Instead, they use disposable toothbrushes in the form of a stem or twig. Pear-tree, lime-tree, currant, raspberry, pine, or spruce would be good choices. Take a pine or spruce twig about 6 inches (15cm) long and chew on one end of it until it resembles a brush. We already achieve a disinfecting effect thanks to some compounds found in evergreen trees. Now we can put our regular toothpaste on the gnawed end, thoroughly brush our teeth, and massage the gums.

I would like to add a few cautionary words about toothpastes. One of the better-known toothpaste manufacturers was recently sued over the high fluoride content in their products resulting in the death of some children who liked to swallow toothpaste as they brushed their teeth. To avoid such tragedy, parents should closely watch their children and stop them from swallowing (many children have this habit). Yoga gurus do not use toothpastes at all. They use powdered salt mixed with oil.

For best effects we should brush our teeth for 3-5 minutes (the average person does it for 30-40 seconds). The Japanese maintain strong and healthy teeth even though they hardly ever use toothbrushes. Instead, they put toothpaste on their index finger and use it to clean their teeth. This is a good way to clean and strengthen the teeth and to massage the gums.

My favorite method is a combination of all methods mentioned above.

Toothpaste preparation: prepare a mixture of one teaspoon of lemon juice, one teaspoon of vegetable oil, two teaspoons of your regular toothpaste, half a teaspoon of baking soda, half a teaspoon of salt, and half a teaspoon of powdered ginger. Stir it well and store in a dark container. Dip your index fingers in the mixture and use them to clean your teeth and massage your gums, 1-2 minutes on each side. Next, brush your teeth for about one minute. Rinse out your mouth thoroughly using plenty of water.

After this, drink a cup of green tea. It prevents tooth decay and destroys microorganisms that damage our tooth enamel.

Tongue cleaning

Our tongue is in most cases covered with whitish or yellowish plaque coating, which indicates digestive tract disorders and unhealthy waste deposits in the body. We should, of course, put our digestive tract in order. The tongue should be cleaned as often as the teeth; we do not want our tongue to be the breeding ground for oral bacteria. The method is very simple: Scrape the plaque off with your index finger moving from the back of the tongue towards its tip until the normal pink coloring shows on the entire surface, then apply some oil.

Nose cleaning

Unfortunately nose cleaning is not as much of a habit with most people as tooth brushing. Many of us put up with all the unpleasant consequences of our nose being plugged up with mucus. This does not only interfere with correct breathing and the sense of smell, but it also creates other health problems by disturbing the energy balance in our body. I covered this topic partially in the previous chapters. Here I would just like to add a few remarks about breathing through nasal passages.

Ancient Chinese medicine regarded breathing through the right side of the nose as solar and positive (increasing the positive charge in the body), while breathing through the left side was called lunar or negative. To maintain the bio-energy balance, we must be able to freely breathe through both sides of our nose.

Dust getting into our nose is trapped in the sticky mucous lining of the nasal passages and is swept out by the movements of microscopic hairs called cilia. Nasal mucous lining has antiseptic qualities and is able to kill a lot of bacteria. The air we breathe contains so much dust that these defense mechanisms and even the use of hygienic tissue are not able to clean it all. In addition, most people sleep on the side (the healthy way to sleep is on the back) and this way one side of their nose accumulates more dust than the other side. This makes normal, even breathing impossible and influences the composition and circulation of our blood. This eventually leads to sleep disorders, nervous system disorders, and digestive problems. People with chronic colds age faster, suffer from vision disorders, and experience buzzing sounds in their head and ears. The inability to breathe evenly through both sides of the nose, in time leads to a general decline of our health. This is why at any age, as part of our daily hygiene, we should clean our nose cavities and air passages by irrigating them with a solution.

Let us take a look at the technique.

Useful advice:

Dissolve two pinches of salt and baking soda and half a teaspoon of honey in half a cup of warm water. Pour the solution in a nursing bottle and cut a bigger opening in the bottle's nipple to let the solution easily get through. Plug one side of your nose with your thumb, put the bottle's nipple in the other nostril and draw the solution until it comes out through your mouth. Repeat the procedure for the other side of your nose. Do it in turns until you use up the solution. When you learn the technique well, you can double the amounts of water and other ingredients. Perform the procedure in the morning or the evening two to three times a week. From time to time you can use half a cup of mint or chamomile extract, for its antiseptic and aromatic qualities.

Nose irrigation stimulates the nerve endings and mucous membrane. It helps maintain adequate level of moisture inside your nose in hot weather. Nose irrigation with seawater is very effective. Based on my experience and the testimony of my patients, I am strongly convinced that nose irrigation is the only effective method against many disorders originating in our nose cavities. It is the best therapy against chronic colds and has a toning effect on our brain and nervous system. **Note:** During nose irrigation with seawater, you are going to experience burning and stinging sensations in your nose at first. This happens because the mucous lining is unhealthy and damaged. These unpleasant sensations will stop after 3-4 irrigations.

Many laryngologists are against nose irrigation – they prescribe nasal drops instead. But patients who dry up the mucous lining of their nose and mouth by the use of drops and still do not get any results are often willing to try this method. What practice proves is often different from what theory teaches. After a few irrigations, the mucous lining of your nose becomes healthy and strong, you can forget about colds, and you are finally able to fully breathe through your nose.

Ear cleaning

Ear hygiene is not very complicated but it is essential for our overall health. Nature provided for periodic ear cleaning by means of earwax. As the secretion comes out of the ear canal, it carries away dust that might have got inside the ear. If earwax does not move along well, it creates pressure on eardrums. This may cause headaches, dizziness, and even loss of hearing. The principle of ear hygiene is simple: We help earwax loosen up by squeezing, twisting, and pulling our ears in different directions. All these movements help the earwax and impurities move along and come out of the ear. It is an excellent idea to include the following ear massage in your daily morning hygienic routine (repeat each movement eight times):

1. Push the humps behind your ears up and down.
2. Bend your ears forward and back.
3. Twist your ears clockwise.
4. Pull down your earlobes.

After this, you can put your index fingers in the ears and move them sidewise in different directions, then remove loose earwax (along with dust and dead cells).

My experience shows that many of my readers are first determined to follow advice and procedures suggested in my books, but eventually they become overwhelmed with their everyday duties and return to their former lifestyle, which does not include much effort aimed at maintaining good health. I want to remind you that you only have one life and you owe it to yourself to stay healthy and use your life to the full potential. All aspects of our health are important. The way our physiology works requires comprehensive care of the entire body.

INTERNAL BODY HYGIENE

We hear from our childhood about external body hygiene, but we know little about internal hygiene. However, the condition of our internal organs determines much of our external appearance.

You have read this information in the first part of my book. I purposely repeat the segment here to help you understand the information better in the context of complete body cleansing.

Not many of us know that a grown person's large intestine contains 17-33 lb (8-15 kg) of hardened fecal material that we carry around all life long. Usually after the age of 40, our large intestine is so full of fecal matter that it crowds out other organs and interferes with the functioning of our liver, kidneys, and lungs. It is a considerable cause of diseases. Let us explain how it works.

Our large intestine is like a pot containing fertile soil in the form of digested food. The body is like a plant. The walls of the large intestine are lined with roots that, like roots of a plant, absorb nutritious substances into our blood. Each group of roots nurtures a specific organ. Useless waste is discarded. What happens with the undigested food?

During the next meal, a new undigested chunk sticks to the old one, then another one. Undigested food sticks to the large intestine's walls. We carry around a few pounds of those chunks. It is not hard to imagine what happens with food products "stored" for many years in temperatures above 96.8F (36C). The intestine still performs its absorbing function under this layer of filth and delivers toxins, carcinogenic substances - products of decay, to the body. Obviously, this is not good material for building healthy cells. Toxins circulate with blood and gradually ruin our health by forming deposits on the walls of blood vessels or in the joints.

Deposits of stagnant fecal matter form hardened layers. The huge sack of waste pushes internal organs out of their proper places, creates pressure on the diaphragm, significantly lowering the capacity of our lungs. The liver is pushed out of its place; there is pressure on the kidneys; the small intestine does not have enough space for its movements; men find their genital-urinary systems crowded. The lower section of the rectum is put under most stress: overworked veins expand and form bloody lumps. A poisoned large intestine can cause countless problems and diagnosis of diseases is unpredictable. In the worst-case scenario, last stages of cancer, the passage of waste in the large intestine is completely blocked and the body dies poisoned by its own toxins.

Large intestine cleansing

Some symptoms of an unclean large intestine: constipation, bloating, skin eczemas, pimples, allergies, black stains on the teeth, gray coating on the tongue, unpleasant skin smell and sweating.

Useful advice:

1. Limit your consumption of meat, chocolate, sweets, sugar, cow milk, eggs, and white bread.
2. Drink one cup of kefir every morning and evening.
3. Chew your food thoroughly (each bite 35-50 times).
4. Do not drink during meals.
5. Drink less coffee and tea.

You can test the functioning of your large intestine the following way: Drink two tablespoons of freshly squeezed beet juice. If after four hours your urine becomes red, your large intestine is not functioning properly.

Enema

I would like to treat the subject of enema (intestinal irrigation) in more detail because enema is one of the most effective procedures you can do at home to clean toxins from your body.

Some specialists warn that large intestine irrigation destroys the healthy microflora. I do not agree with that. It is almost impossible to find a person with a healthy microflora because of our diet, lack of exercise, and the amount of medications (especially antibiotics) we take. I would guess that about 90% of people have a degenerated digestive tract and a damaged microflora. Dr. Norman Walker, an American physician known around the world (he lived for 106 years) used enema for 50 years to treat different diseases. He regarded enema to be the simplest and most effective method to clean internal filth from the body. He used to say that people who do not believe in enema's effectiveness need it most.

Practice shows that many people are not ready to use the large intestine irrigation routine because it seems repulsive to them. They should realize that it is the only way to remove layers of stagnant fecal matter accumulated in their intestine. Stagnant matter looks much more repulsive, and its smell is worse than the worst sewage system smell you can imagine. Other people find the position inconvenient or do not have enough space at home to perform the procedure. There are many excuses. But the threat of an operation or death provides an instant motivation to try putting their large intestine in order. The most reasonable behavior is to start using the procedure before we are faced with any serious health threats.

Before I start describing the procedure in detail, I would like you to remember two things. First, your motivation can be provided by the desire to get rid of stagnant deposits that cause many health problems. Second, you must follow the prescribed routine in detail to avoid harming yourself and to achieve maximum benefits.

The technique of enema – large intestine irrigation

Make a solution of 1.5-2 quarts (1.5-2L) of boiled water (at body temperature) and 1-2 tablespoons of lemon juice (filter pulp and seeds out of the juice). Put the solution in the enema bag (available in most pharmacies).

Hang the bag about 3-5ft (1-1.5m) above your body level; apply some vegetable oil to the enema tubing and your anus. Vegetable oil is preferred to vaseline, creams, or soap because it is a natural product and does not plug up skin pores. Assume the "tiger position" – down on your knees and elbows, your legs slightly spread, your abdomen relaxed as much as possible. Insert the end of the tubing into your anus and let water flow into it. Breathe deeply through the open mouth. The enema bag will be empty in 1-2 minutes and then you can get up. (If water does not flow freely from the bag, squeeze the enema tube to stop the flow completely for a few seconds and then let the water flow again.)

This is not the end of the procedure. You should shake up your intestine a little. One of the ways to do it is to do some jumping and shaking of the lower abdomen with your hands. In any way, try to create some washing action inside your intestine, then lie on your back and wait. You will feel a bowel movement reflex in 2-10 minutes. Be prepared to spend 15-20 minutes on the toilet – take a magazine or a book to read. Eventually you will feel that all water has left your large intestine (urination is the final sign).

If you are new to the procedure, it is a good idea to take a look at the waste washed out with water. The sight is unpleasant, even repulsive, but this is what it takes to provide strong motivation for the future.

The routine should be repeated every day in the first week, every second day in the second and third week, and twice in the fourth week.

After the fourth week, most of you will know by the look and smell of your stools that the cleaning has been successful. To maintain your large intestine in this clean state from then on, it is enough to perform the routine once a week for the rest of your life.

What you have just done can be compared to cleaning up soil around your body's "roots" by removing layers of hardened fecal matter, mold, putrefaction and fermentation products. Now these roots can absorb useful substances from the digested food, needed to build new cells. Your body absorbs no more harmful and carcinogenic toxins. Now your blood can be cleansed and the development of diseases reversed. You have achieved it all by yourself.

All organs can receive better nutrition, and clean blood is able to dissolve harmful deposits in other parts of the body. Internal organs gradually return to their proper places, their functioning improves, blood pressure normalizes from day to day, and no diseases affect your body anymore.

Our large intestine that has been stretched, withered, and malnourished for a long time has to be returned to its proper shape in order to efficiently perform its important functions. When it is returned to the natural shape, it learns again to move along the masses of undigested food and other waste.

In order to achieve this, we can eat a lot of grains during the weeks of our enema therapy (it is a good idea at any time). Make sure it is whole grains. Use only water to prepare them. As a grain meal passes through the stomach, small intestine, and then enters the large

185

intestine, it helps the large intestine assume the proper shape.
Note: Just remember not to use any milk in preparing your grains.
I presented Dr. Walker's intestinal irrigation as the simplest and most effective method of cleaning up layers of hardened feces from your large intestine. There are a few more notes I would like to add:

1. Many people are concerned at first with the amount of water used in the procedure 1.5-2 quarts (1.5-2L). The capacity of our large intestine (clean and healthy) is about 3.5 quarts (3.5L) – you still have some spare room left. The feelings of discomfort cannot be avoided at first but they cease eventually. In the future, when the intestine is clean, it is enough to use just 1 quart (1L) of solution for prevention.
2. Why do we add lemon juice? Alkaline environment promotes fermentation and putrefaction processes. By introducing mild acidity, we slow down these reactions, destroy disease-causing bacteria, and stimulate the development of friendly healthy microflora. Acidic lemon juice destroys toxins and mold (mold is flushed out with water in the form of dark threads.)

For those who find the procedure unacceptable because of its nature, I would like to present a few alternative methods of large intestine cleansing. You should remember, however, that they are not as effective as enema.

Using kefir, apple juice, and vegetable salads to cleanse the large intestine

Day one: drink 2.5 quarts (2.5L) of kefir (in 6 doses) and eat dark grain biscuits (do not eat anything else all day).
Day two: drink 1.5-2 quarts (1.5-2L) of apple juice (in 6 portions) and eat only dark grain biscuits all day. The juice should be freshly squeezed out of sweet apples.
Day three: eat only vegetable salads (cooked beets, carrots, potatoes with added pickled cucumbers, sauerkraut, onion, vegetable oil) and dark grain biscuits.
Use this therapy twice a month.

Using fruits to cleanse large intestine

1. Grind up 14oz (400g) of dried plums, 7oz (200g) of dates, 7oz (200g) of apricots, and 7oz (200g) of figs. Add 7oz (200g) of honey and blend well. Store refrigerated in a glass container. Take one tablespoon before going to bed every night until finished. Use the therapy once every three months.
2. Peel 2 oranges (leave the white lining on the fruits). Eat the fruits two hours after your last meal, 14 nights in a row.
3. Put 10 dried plums in a cup filled with buttermilk, let them soak overnight, drink the buttermilk and eat the fruits on an empty stomach in the morning. In the same way, soak ten dried plums all day, drink the buttermilk, and eat the plums before going to bed at night. Repeat the routine for at least ten days. Use once every three months.

Many ill people still fear the irrigation procedure and want to use laxatives for intestinal cleansing. I definitely discourage the use of laxatives. They dry up the intestines and cause dehydration of our entire body. Our large intestine's muscles should be made to work. Laxatives cause the emptying of the intestine without engaging the muscle tissue, which leads to its weakening. Weak intestinal muscles, in turn, cause chronic constipation. Enema, in contrast, stimulates and normalizes our large intestine's function. People who went through a series of enemas do not suffer from constipation.

To bring the expected results, all cleansing routines have to be done in the appropriate order. You just learned about the first step – large intestine cleansing. There is no other way to start complete body cleansing. If you try to skip it and go ahead with the other routines, they will not produce results.

This may be better understood in the context of another secret to maintaining good health: For best results, internal hygiene must go together with smart nutrition. You will be fully protected from any diseases by applying this principle. Intestinal cleaning itself does not protect us from huge energy losses in the process of digesting improperly combined meals. Similarly, a proper diet will not stop deadly toxins accumulated in our large intestine from being absorbed in the blood stream. On the contrary, it stimulates the absorbing functions. There is only one way to go – cleansing has to be done by performing the whole presented set of routines.

Having completed the intestinal cleansing cycle, we should learn about the proper combining of foods (Use Table 2, page 103) and help our large intestine in building a healthy microflora.

Building up a healthy intestinal microflora

By frequent use of medications (especially antibiotics), eating sweets and yeasted baked goods, drinking milk, and improperly combining foods, we make it possible for unfriendly microorganisms (bacteria, fungi, yeast) to breed in our digestive tract. These parasites grow into our mucous membrane, feed on our blood, and excrete toxic physiological products. The toxins bring us headaches; fatigue; colds; frequent eye, bladder, and kidney inflammations; strong pains in our stomach, liver, etc. The problems caused by the unfriendly microorganisms are quite unpredictable. They cause dysbacteriosis - (degeneration of intestinal microflora). The best remedy against these disease-causing parasites is garlic.

Not too much of a good thing

Garlic is a natural antibiotic. As any medicine, it has to be taken accordingly to accurately prescribed doses. This is why earlier described therapy (page 91) and the one described below use only small amounts of garlic.

I believe that normally two to three garlic cloves a week in addition to the amount that we consume with our salads and other foods is the adequate intake. The therapy needed for rebuilding healthy intestinal microflora requires increased amounts of garlic

As a therapy, eat one garlic clove every evening, two hours after supper, for two weeks. Remember to chew your garlic well and take it without bread. This may cause a strong burning sensation in your mouth, throat, and stomach. It is necessary to undergo this suffering - as garlic juice kills disease-causing bacteria, it penetrates small abrasions where the parasites breed. People with circulatory disorders can get an increased heartbeat. It is natural because garlic is the only product containing dissolved germanium - an element that wonderfully cleanses and regenerates blood vessels. All these slight inconveniences are worth suffering for the sake of your health. You can rinse out your mouth, brush your teeth, have a tea with lemon and honey, or eat an apple before bedtime to remove the garlic smell. Other ways to do it would be chewing on a lemon peel, orange peel, or cut up parsley. People who find it impossible to chew a garlic clove can cut it in half and swallow like pills or take the clove with a bread coating around it to reduce the burning sensation.

Having done the intestinal cleansing, we can turn attention to our body's "chemical laboratory," which is our liver. It has an important part in the speedy regeneration of our health.

Liver cleansing

Some external symptoms of an unclean liver

1. Freckles, brown moles, and warts on the skin
2. Brown stains around hair roots
3. Cold and moist skin on the body and hands
4. Yellow stains on the bottom of the tongue
5. Walking in uneven steps

Causes of poor liver function:

- Excessive consumption of food and fluids
- Too much sugar, sweets, fruits, and alcohol
- Too much animal fat, fatty meat, and vegetable oil in the diet
- Eating mainly cooked and refined food products
- Too much fresh bread and other flour-based products
- The habit of eating before bedtime or at night

Useful advice:

1. Limit the number of meals and snacks.
2. Do not eat breakfast.
3. Eat more steamed vegetables (30-40% of the diet).
4. Eat more sauerkraut in the winter.
5. Eat more cottage cheese, kefir, and buttermilk.
6. Eat only freshly prepared meals (do not store and warm them up).
7. Try to use water from melted ice (see earlier chapters) for your cooking and drinking

Liver cleansing should be followed by gallbladder cleansing and pancreas cleansing.

The liver is one of our most important internal organs. It is our body's "chemical laboratory," and its functioning influences the condition of our heart, circulatory system, digestive organs, kidneys, brain, and lymphatic system; it also influences our psychological wellbeing. Most people who eat improperly combined meals have their liver partially filled with stones, particles of cholesterol and bilirubin (waste from the breakdown of red blood cells that were not removed from the body for various reasons) as early as at the age of five.

There are many formulas that can improve the functioning of our liver, but none of them brings results that would be as obvious as the results of a cleansing procedure. People who had been suffering from gallstones for more than ten years and were supposed to go through a surgery took care of the problem once and for all by cleansing their liver. There was no need for the surgery anymore.

There are many cases where a bad condition of the liver disturbs the functioning of the heart.

I would like to mention one such case from my natural therapy practice. A 36-year-old female patient had a heart disease, looked pale and skinny, suffered from breathing problems, and could not walk. Her doctors had suggested an operation: removing part of her aorta and replacing it with a segment taken from her iliac artery. She had been warned that such an operation has the success rate of only 30-40%. She came to our therapy center looking for help. We diagnosed a fairly significant inefficiency in the functioning of her liver. What would be the point of an operation if the blood in her veins remained contaminated, thick, and acidic? Even if the operation were successful, her health would return to the same condition in five to seven years. A transplant would remove the symptoms but would not remove the real cause – the poor quality of her blood. Once the blood is clean, the system that delivers it will heal as well.

The woman received the large intestine cleansing procedure and three routines of liver cleansing. In three months, she appeared to be a totally different person – healthy, joyous, and optimistic.

Many people are naive in their belief that there cannot be anything wrong with their liver. From my own experience and that of my patients', I know that such assumption is a big mistake. Bile stones stick very hard to the liver. There were no stones removed in the woman's first and second cleansing, only dark green cholesterol particles and pieces of mold looking like fragments of a spider web. However, the third cleansing produced half a jar of stones, a lot of old bile, dark flakes and other filth. Everybody's liver has this kind of filth in it, and the amount increases when we get older. Getting rid of it makes us feel lighter and rejuvenates our entire body. Liver cleansing is as natural and necessary as periodic cleaning of your home.

Based on my own experience and that of other natural therapy specialists, I am fully convinced that liver-cleansing procedure causes no side effects as long as all <u>instructions are followed in detail.</u>

Instructions for liver cleansing

Note: The effect of the cleansing routine depends on following these instructions in detail and completing all stages of the procedure.

Stage 1 – Preparation for cleansing, relaxing the body.

The relaxing effect can be achieved by using the sauna or steam room or hot showers. There should be at least two relaxing sessions (5-7 days before the cleansing). The objective is to warm up, loosen up the body, and generally relax. The last such routine should be done one day before the main cleansing procedure.

Stage 2

Eat mainly plant-based foods 2-3 days before the procedure. Eliminate all kinds of meat and fish from your diet. The only animal products allowed are eggs, kefir, plain yogurt, buttermilk and cottage cheese.

Stage 3

The procedure is best done towards the end of the week (Friday night – Saturday morning or Saturday night – Sunday morning).

Supplies needed:

- 7.5 fl oz (225 ml) of plant oil of any kind (my choice is grape seed oil) – will make 5 drinking portions

191

- 6 average-sized lemons (about 2.2lb/1kg)
- one clove of garlic
- Two small 1.8 fl oz (50ml) cups-glass or plastic (one for oil and one for lemon juice)
- A thermaphore (electric heating pad) or electric pillow
- A jar with a lid

The procedure takes two days.

Day 1

- Eat your last meal before 2 p.m.
- Do not eat any snacks after 2 p.m.
- When you feel hungry, drink fluids (freshly squeezed carrot juice, apple juice, or boiled water are best).
- Most of all, try not to feel tense. You experience weakness because, as your body is cleansing, in absence of food it absorbs some of its toxins. You can help by walking as much as possible or doing other physical activity. Wear warm clothes to prevent loss of energy. In case of headaches or weakness in the evening, immediately perform an enema. If it does not help, drink one cup of hot boiled water with a teaspoon of honey and a teaspoon of apple cider vinegar. Use painkillers only as a last resort.
- Before going to bed, necessarily do an enema. Use about 6 cups (1.5 liter) of water with 0.5 tablespoon of lemon juice.

Day 2

- On awakening, you can drink (in small sips) a glass of hot boiled water.
- Do an enema 1.5 quarts (1.5L) of water, 0.5 tablespoon of lemon juice) and go for a walk.
- You can drink juices before 2 p.m. (carrot, apple, or blended).
- Unhook your phone after 2 p.m.; do not do any household chores or work-related duties. Avoid any unpleasant conversations or stressful situations; try to cut out any interactions.
- Lie down a few times for 20-30 minutes between 3 p.m. and 6 p.m. Try to relax, think of the most pleasant moments of your

life. Warm up your liver with a thermaphore pad or electric pillow (your liver is on the right side, about one inch below your rib cage).

- At 6 p.m. put the bottle with oil into a pot with hot water to slowly warm the oil up.
- Put six lemons into boiling water for 10-15 minutes to make them juicier.
- In the meantime, squeeze juice from one garlic clove into a jar, cover it with a lid and put aside.
- Cut the lemons in half, squeeze them and strain the juice.
- Prepare the bed sheets you will be using during the procedure.

At 6:30 p.m. you should have the following things ready:

- Two 1.8 fl oz (50ml) cups (one for oil and one for lemon juice)
- Electric pillow or a thermaphore pad
- Oil 7.5 fl oz (225ml)
- Lemon juice 5 fl oz (150ml)

At 6:30 p.m. take a ten-minute hot shower, warm your entire body well and lie down.

Make sure to exactly follow all steps of the following schedule from now on:

- Get up at 7 p.m.; pour oil in one cup (1.5 fl oz / 45ml) and lemon juice in the other cup (1 fl oz / 30ml).
- Drink the oil and immediately follow it with lemon juice.
- Lie down again and warm up your liver.
- At 7:15 p.m. get up, drink oil (1.5 fl oz / 45ml) and lemon juice (1 fl oz /30ml), lie down and warm your liver.
- Repeat every 15 minutes until all oil and lemon juice are used up. When you experience nausea (usually after the fourth portion), open the jar with garlic and sniff it. If nausea persists, stop drinking at that stage. Lie down on your right side, put the electric pillow on your liver and do some reading or watch TV.
- Your most unpleasant time will be between 9 p.m. and 11 p.m. You can experience heartburn, weakness, and sweating. You must suffer this discomfort for the sake of your health. People

with a poorly functioning liver might feel their liver "breathe"(a gentle squirting sensation in the area of the right rib cage).

- Do not be afraid. Imagine that you can talk to your liver. Apologize to your liver for the inconvenience. Think that you have been understood and forgiven. This should help your body calm down.
- Limit your walking as much as possible between 9 p.m. and midnight – spend most of the time lying down.
- When you feel bowel movement (about 1 a.m.), go to the toilet. After the stool, perform an enema and go to sleep. In some cases, the bowel movement does not take place until morning. If it does not come till 3 a.m., go to sleep. Your liver cleansing will be completed when you wake up.

Our bodies have their individual qualities. Follow the directions and, at the same time, watch your body's reaction and use your own judgment.

A few further remarks about liver cleansing

1. Some people vomit after their third or fourth portion of oil. This is a sign that their stomach needs to be clean first. It usually happens during the first cleansing. If it happens to you, do not get discouraged. Complete the procedure and wait for results.
2. Try to stay calm and relaxed during the entire procedure. If your liver has a lot of impurities to remove, you might feel it go through movements as if it were breathing. Do not get scared because fear causes spasms in the bile duct and may also cause vomiting.
3. Some people may feel tired the morning after the procedure. The feeling should go away by the evening. In most cases, people have more energy, strength, and zest for life as they get up in the morning.
4. If the liver area feels heavy the next morning, the procedure should be repeated in two weeks.
5. People whose gallbladder has been surgically removed often ask if they can use the procedure. Yes, they can and they need it even more than other people.

6. I tried to include as much detail as possible while describing the procedure because it is like having a small surgery without a scalpel. You have to be well organized and psychologically prepared.
7. If you experience weakness or nausea from drinking oil, from time to time smell the garlic juice you have prepared earlier.

I would like to quickly sum up the main steps of the procedure:

Day 1

- Don't eat anything after 2 p.m. Drink carrot or apple juice – limit the amount to half a glass at a time
- Perform an enema in the evening.

Day 2

- Perform an enema in the morning.
- You can drink juices before 2 p.m.
- Warm up your liver between 3 p.m. and 5 p.m.
- Take a shower at 6:30 p.m.
- At 7 p.m., 7:15, 7:30, 7:45, and 8:00 drink (1.5 fl oz / 45ml) of oil followed by (1 fl oz / 30ml) of lemon juice.
- Warm up your liver between 8 p.m. and 11 p.m. Try to limit your walking as much as possible.
- After the bowel movement between 1 a.m. and 3 a.m., perform an enema.
- Perform another enema on awakening in the morning.
- Eat a light breakfast (fruits and vegetables, other plant-based products, grains). You can have a vegetable soup for dinner, baked or cooked potatoes with green vegetable salad or rice and steamed vegetables for supper, etc. Starting the next day, gradually expand your menu.

How many times can we cleanse our liver?

The first cleansing is the most difficult and uses the most of our body's energy. It usually removes a lot of old bile, mold, white threads, and green swabs – it does not always remove stones. The absence of stones does not mean that the procedure is unsuccessful. It only means that the liver has a lot of impurities in it – the stones will come out in subsequent cleansing procedures. The second cleansing is easier. It should be done 3-4 weeks later and the next ones every three months. There should be 4-7 procedures done in the first year. From then on, continue with just one cleansing a year. You may wonder why the first four procedures are done with such short intervals. The liver has four parts and the first procedure cleanses the first part, the second procedure cleanses the second part, and so on. If you change your diet, subsequent procedures will remove more and more stones. The stones accumulated over many years, became round (like stones on the seashore) and adapted their shapes to the shape of the bile duct. This is why they do not always cause pain but still interfere with your liver's normal functioning. A cleansing procedure first breaks the stones up, moves them, and causes them to change shapes. Subsequent procedures can easily remove the stones.

The word "stones" does not accurately describe the material we are talking about. They are really soft clay-like chunks the size of a pea, a bean, or sometimes a walnut.

The diet after liver cleansing

You should limit the consumption of products that can damage your liver. They are: fried meat, spicy fat snacks (especially cold), starch foods such as white flour, cakes, and sweet biscuits. If your liver is ill, limit vinegar, pepper, mustard, turnips, radish, fried onion, coffee, and tea. To strengthen your ill liver, you can drink a blend of beet juice and carrot juice (proportion 1:4), up to 0.5 quarts (0.5L) a day. Vitamins that are essential for your liver (A, C, B, K) are found in large amounts in egg yolk, butter, cottage cheese, tomatoes, beets, carrot, squash, cauliflower, grapes, watermelon, strawberries, apples, dried plums, wheat sprouts, wild rose, and currant.

Useful advice:

There is a very effective remedy against inflammations of the liver and gallbladder: grind 3.5oz (100g) sprouting wheat, 3.5oz (100g) cooked beets, 3.5oz (100g) cooked carrots, and 3.5oz (100g) dried apricot. Add 2 tablespoons of lemon juice and some honey. The blend should have a pleasant sour taste. You can add some butter or vegetable oil (always add them to your ready meals – do not use for cooking or frying).

Using vegetable juices for liver cleansing

The presented above method of liver cleansing with the use of oil and lemon juice is the most effective; however, some people are not able to drink oil, they cannot even stand its smell. What can they do about it? They can cleanse their liver with vegetable juice blends. This method is longer and less effective.

Drink half a glass of carrot, beet, and cucumber juice blend 3-4 times everyday in proportion 10:3:3 e.g. 8.8oz: 2.6oz: 2.6oz (250g: 75g: 75g) for two weeks. Perform this 14-day therapy four times (every three months) in the first year and once a year from then on.

Liver cleansing with apple juice

Apple juice works wonders at cleansing our body, especially liver, kidneys, and gallbladder.
Use only freshly squeezed juice (store bought juices do not bring the expected results). Use mostly sweet apples – add just a few from a sour variety to achieve a pleasant taste. Drink in small sips and hold each sip in your mouth for a while to let it blend with your saliva. People with unhealthy digestive tract microflora can suffer from some stomach discomfort, such as bloating, after drinking the juice. To prevent the discomfort, they can filter the remaining pulp particles from the juice. You can earlier prepare your digestive system to be able to handle high acid content by drinking half a glass of apple juice 15 minutes before every meal during the proceeding week. The cleansing lasts three days. You have to abstain from any food. Outdoor physical activity would be beneficial.

Each day of the procedure, drink only apple juice in the following amounts:

- 8 a.m. – 1 glass
- 10 a.m. – 1 glass
- 12 noon – 2 glasses
- 2 p.m. – 2 glasses
- 4 p.m. – 2 glasses
- 6 p.m. – 1 glass
- 8 p.m. – 1 glass

If there is no bowel movement during the therapy, you can drink stool-stimulating herbal beverages or, even better, perform an enema.

Bone and joint cleansing

It is hard to meet a person who would not suffer from some kind of bone and joint pain. It makes no difference for the afflicted what we call the illness: rheumatism, arthritis, or osteoporosis. The label does not change the pain. I have met many suffering people in the course of my practice. There were children, youth, and middle-aged people among them. I feel most for the elderly because they are unhappy and helpless like nobody else. They do not catch our attention because they are not seen in the streets very much. In most cases, they spend a lot of time at home alone with their pain. Most of them are already tired of life. Sleepless nights and limited mobility result in sad voice and tired-looking eyes. The common view is that people are lucky if they are still alive at the age of seventy. It does not bring much comfort to hear words such as, "it's hard to be old but don't worry since you can't do anything about it." Younger people use such phrases without thinking that, before they know it, they will be in the same position and will be offered the same kind of comfort.

Ancient Tibetan wisdom teaches: "Strong bones and flexible joints assure long and healthy life."

There are many factors that influence the condition of our bones and joints. Diet and the level of physical activity are two examples. We have a large degree of control over these two factors and must remember to make good choices. There is one factor that nobody can fully control – our aging.

No matter how much we care about our internal hygiene, toxic salty deposits will always form on our bones and joints. They limit our joints' range of motion and cause painful inflammations (rheumatism, arthritis, etc.). One of the ways to avoid these diseases is regular cleansing of bones and joints.

One stage of the therapy takes three consecutive days and uses 15g of bay leaves.

Day 1 – Break up 0.18oz (5g) of bay leaves, put in 10 fl oz (300 ml) of boiling water, and boil slowly for 5 minutes. Pour into a thermos and put aside for 5 hours to settle. Strain it into another container and drink in small sips every 15-20 minutes over 12 hours.

Note: Never drink the entire extract at one time – this could cause a hemorrhage.

Day 2 and 3 – Continue as on the first day.

During the therapy eliminate meat, eggs, cheese, cottage cheese, etc. from your menu.

As salts and sand are excreted during the therapy, your urine's color may change to any from green to light red. This is a normal phenomenon. **It is a two-stage therapy with a seven-day interval and it should be used once a year.** The best time to undergo this therapy is the summer-fall season.

Kidney cleansing

Some external symptoms of unclean kidneys:

1. Bags under the eyes
2. White spots on the nails
3. Moist palms

Some causes of poor kidney function:

- Accumulation of mucus and the formation of stones
- Widening of kidneys due to high fluid intake
- Shrinking of kidneys as a result of excessive consumption of salt, meat, fish, breads, sweets, flour-based and refined products

199

Bags under the eyes are a symptom of excess fluids or fat deposits in the kidneys. If the bags are soft, the fluid intake is too high. Hard bags under the eyes mean too high consumption of fat dairy products, animal fats and fatty meat, and sweets. Red eyelids signal the formation of kidney stones.

With well-functioning kidneys, we urinate 3-4 times a day. If urination is more frequent, we should limit our fluid intake. The color of urine should resemble light beer. Very light coloring means we need more salt; if the color is too dark, we should limit our salt intake.

Another sign that the salt intake is too high is dark brown rings around the eyes. In such a case, we have to eliminate salt from our diet and use other kinds of seasoning (dried garlic, parsley, etc.).

Out of many available kidney-cleansing methods, I am going to describe four most effective ones. Please choose one that suits you best. Regardless of the chosen method, you should eliminate high-protein foods from your menu for the time of the therapy, in particular: liver, fried and smoked meat, salted fish, meat soups, etc. Eat more salads, fruits, and sprouting wheat. You can use some salt in your salads to stimulate the kidneys. Avoid sweets because they interfere with your kidneys' proper functioning.

Method 1

This method is identical to the described earlier liver-cleansing method with vegetable juices or apple juice.

Method 2

For good kidney-cleansing results, drink half a glass of carrot, celery, and parsley juice blend (proportion 9:5:2) 3-4 times a day for two weeks. Use this therapy once a year during the summer-fall season.

Method 3

Wild rose fruit brew is helpful in dissolving all stones in the body and reducing them to sand. Boil 2 tablespoons of wild rose fruits in 7 fl oz (200ml) of water for 15 minutes, let it cool off, and strain the brew. Drink 1/3 of a glass three times a day for two weeks. Repeat the therapy every three months.

Method 4

Parsnip juice is a very effective remedy against genital-urinary system disorders and kidney stones (especially when there is protein in the urine or the kidneys are infected). It is a strong remedy and should be taken separately (best on empty stomach), in its pure form, 1.1-1.8oz (30-50g) once a day from October to January.

After we get rid of kidney stones, we should, first of all, make changes in our diet. The stones are only a symptom. The main cause of their formation is excess of uric acid and its salts in our body due to a high-protein diet, inactive lifestyle, etc.

Lymph and blood cleansing of radioactive and toxic compounds
(especially useful after chemotherapy)

This therapy should be used at the beginning of the season for flu and other infectious epidemics. You can quickly and effectively prevent infections in your body without any antibiotics. Use 2.2 quarts (2.2L) of juice blend daily. Prepare fresh blend every day.

The content of the blend for one day (freshly squeezed juices only) should be as follows: 32oz/900g of grapefruit juice, 32oz/900g of orange juice, 7oz/200g of lemon juice, and 7oz/200g of distilled water. The therapy lasts three days (do not eat anything except oranges or grapefruits).

Drink a solution of one teaspoon of bitter salt (epsom salt) in a glass of warm water on an empty stomach in the morning. Dress warmly and drink half a glass of fruit juice blend every 30 minutes until the entire blend is finished. The procedure helps remove toxic deposits from all parts of the body. The solution attracts toxins from the lymph just like a magnet attracts iron. The toxic wastes are gathered in the intestines and are discarded. The body is dehydrated in the process and you need to drink the fast-absorbable juice blend to replenish the fluids.

When you feel hungry, eat oranges or grapefruits and nothing else. There may be heavy sweating during the procedure – this is one of the normal ways your body is removing impurities.

The second and third days are the same as the first. The therapy should be used once a year, in the early spring or late fall.

Circulatory system cleansing
(blood vessels and veins)

Put 1 cup of Fennel seeds, 2 tablespoons of ground valerian roots, and 2 cups of natural honey into a 2-quart (2L) pot. Pour 1 quart (1L) of boiled water on it, heat up slowly, and boil for 2 minutes. Set aside and keep at room temperature for 10 hours. You can cover it with a towel to keep the heat in. Strain the liquid and keep in the refrigerator. Take 1 tablespoon 3 times a day, 30 minutes before mealtime, until finished. Use this therapy once a year.

Additional methods of internal body cleansing

So far I presented the basic methods of internal body cleansing. There are certain additional procedures that help to thoroughly clean up every little corner of our body.

Honey enema

Dissolve 1 tablespoon of honey in a glass of water at room temperature and add 1 tablespoon of lemon juice. Use 1-2 times a month as your enema solution.

Coffee enema

Put 3 tablespoons of ground coffee into 7 fl oz (200ml) of boiling water and boil for 3 minutes. Lower the heat and brew for another 12 minutes. Strain it and let it cool off to room temperature. Coffee enema has enormous benefits – it stimulates the lining of the large intestine and removes toxins from it. It also wonderfully stimulates the functioning of the liver and gallbladder. Unlike the coffee we drink, it does not damage the nervous system, flush out calcium, or destroy group B vitamins. The therapy can be used once a month.

Liver cleansing

People often ask me questions about liver cleansing methods for the elderly or children, alternative to the procedures described above.

The methods presented so far might not suit some people, for example not everybody can live on just juices for two days or drink 7 fl oz (200ml) of oil (especially in the case of children). I would like to describe an alternative method for them. It is a little complicated so please pay close attention to the method, especially the amounts of ingredients used.

Liver cleansing for the elderly and children (without the use of oil)

Sets #1 and #2 are to be prepared at the same time (within one hour).

Set #1
Grind 3 cups of oats and put it in an enamel 5-quart (5L) pot, then pour 4 quarts (4L) of cold water on it. Cover the pot with a lid and set aside for 24 hours.

Set #2
Take a cup of wild rose fruit, chop them into small pieces, put in a 2-quart (2L) pot, and pour 1 quart (1L) of boiling water on it. Wrap the pot with a towel and set it aside for 24 hours.

After 24 hours, add 2 tablespoons of birch buds and 3 tablespoons of raspberry leaves to the pot with oat and boil it for 15 minutes. Add 2 tablespoons of corn fibers (found under corn leaves) and slowly boil for another 15 minutes. Set the brew aside for 45 minutes to settle and carefully strain it.

Strain set #2 and blend both sets. The resulting blend is a liver-cleansing remedy for an adult.

If you want to prepare a liver-cleansing blend for a child, reduce the amounts of ingredients according to the age of the child by the following factors:

- Age 1-3 – 10 times
- Age 4-6 – 8 times
- Age 7-10 – 6 times
- Age 11-15 – 4 times

Pour the blend into bottles and store in the refrigerator or any dry, dark, and cool place. Take 5.1 fl oz (150ml) four times a day, half an hour before meals (try to limit yourself to four small meals a day). The last time you take the blend should not be later than 7 p.m.

Use the following amounts for children (four times a day):

- Age 1-3 – one teaspoon for two weeks
- Age 3-5 – two teaspoons for two weeks
- Age 5-7 – one tablespoon for two weeks
- Age 7-10 – two tablespoons for two weeks
- Age 10-15 – four tablespoons for two weeks
- Over 15 – 5.1 fl oz / 150ml until the blend is finished

Use the therapy once a year.

Kidney cleansing

Method A – Using parsnips and celery roots

Take 2.2lb (1kg) of parsnips and 1.1lb (0.5kg) of celery roots, clean them, rinse, and grind up. Put the grinds in a 4-5 quart (4-5 L) pot; add 2.2lb/1kg of honey and 1 quart (1L) of cool boiled water. Using low heat and stirring with a wooden spoon, bring to the point of boiling, then cover with a lid and put in the refrigerator for 3 days. On the forth day, add 1 quart (1L) of boiled water, slowly heat up to the point of boiling, let it cool off a little and strain it. Pour this syrup into bottles and store in a dark place. Take 3 tablespoons twice a day 15 minutes before meals until the syrup is used up.

Method B – Using currant

Take 3 tablespoons of young currant leaves, pour 0.5 quart (0.5 L) of boiling water on them, set aside for 20 minutes, squeeze out the leaves and discard them. Slowly heat up the brew almost to the point of boiling, add 2 tablespoons of fresh, frozen, or dried currant, and set aside for 3 hours. Drink in small sips throughout the day half a glass at a time and eat the currant fruits. This method can be used throughout the year not only for its kidney-cleansing effect but also as a rich source of vitamins.

Circulatory system cleansing

The remedies described below are effective against circulatory system disorders – they lower the cholesterol level, reduce high blood pressure, stop buzzing noises in the head and ears, and improve vision.

Squeeze juice from 0.8lb (350g) of cleaned garlic and 24 lemons; blend both juices and put the blend in the refrigerator for 24 hours. Take 1 teaspoon of the blend followed by half a glass of kefir, buttermilk, or plain yogurt every day before bedtime until the blend is used up.

Blood cleansing (1)

Pour 0.5 cup of boiling water over 1 tablespoon of green tea leaves, let it stand for 10 minutes, add whole (non pasteurized, organic, best from the farm) milk to fill the glass, add a pinch of salt, and stir. Drink the blend on an empty stomach in the morning. Use the same recipe in the evening but add a teaspoon of honey instead of a pinch of salt. Drink before bedtime, at least two hours after your last meal. Repeat the routine for six days. Perform an enema before bedtime every other day. Eat plant-based food (vegetables, grains, bread, oil) during the therapy.

Blood cleansing (2)

Blend 3.4 fl oz (100ml) of nettle juice (squeezed from May and June nettle) with 3.4 fl oz (100ml) of sugar-free apple juice (can be store-bought) and drink on an empty stomach 30 minutes before breakfast. Use the therapy for 20 days, make a 10-day interval, and follow by another 20 days.

Thyroid gland cleansing

Cut up 40 apple seeds and pour 3.4 fl oz (100ml) of vodka (40% proof and up) over it. Let it stand for 7 days in a dark place. Take 7 drops diluted in 0.7 fl oz (20ml) of water 15 minutes before meals. Use the therapy once every three months. You can use 21 grapefruit seeds instead of 40 apple seeds.

Cleansing the respiratory organs

The therapy can be used by smokers and people suffering from disorders of respiratory passages.

Method A

Wash and peel a black radish, cut it up and run through a juicer. Add 1 tablespoon of honey and drink before bedtime. Put the pulp on a cotton sheet and use as a compress on your chest (except the heart area). Cover the compress with a towel or blanket. Take the compress off in the case of a strong burning sensation to avoid damage to the skin. Rub some vegetable oil on your chest.

Method B - Cabbage compress

Take four white cabbage leaves (large enough to cover your lung area), put them in a pot with water, bring to the point of boiling, and cook for exactly 3 minutes. Rub some lard on your chest and back in the lungs area, use 2 leaves to cover your chest and 2 to cover your back. Wrap a towel around it, put on a warm shirt, and cover yourself with a warm blanket. Repeat this for three evenings before bedtime. After the second day, your lungs will start releasing phlegm; there will be coughing and heavy sweating (this is a normal phenomenon).

Method C - Using pine sap

Warm up a cup of goat milk (do not boil) and put a piece of pine tree resin in it. Stir to dissolve the sap completely and let the mixture cool off a little. Drink it warm before bedtime, rub some herbal warming balsam on your chest and back, and put on a warm shirt.

Cleansing the eyes (lenses)

Methods described below help remove lens clouding due to cataracts.

Method A

Pour 2 cups of boiling water over 2 teaspoons of Marigold flowers, let it stand for 30 minutes, and strain it. Drink half a glass 3 times a day, preferably 15-20 minutes before meals. Use the remaining brew to make eye compresses in the evening and the morning, 5-10 minutes each time. Repeat the routine for one month.

Method B - Using sunlight to cleanse the eyes

To improve your vision and prevent vision disorders, you can look at the Sun with wide-open eyes before 8 a.m. and after 6 p.m. (especially in April and May). The duration of each therapy session should be as follows:

- Week 1 - 1 minute
- Week 2 - 2 minutes
- Week 3 - 3 minutes
- Week 4 - 5 minutes

If your eyes start hurting, look in the general direction of the Sun instead of looking straight at it.

Using black radish for body cleansing

(Joints, lymphatic system, circulatory system, and other internal organs)

Take 22lb (10kg) of black radish, wash them well, cut out all fibers and unhealthy spots without peeling, and then grind them up. Put the grinds through a juicer - you will get about 3 quarts (3L) of juice. Pour the juice into glass bottles, close the bottles, and store in the refrigerator (**Note:** This is important - do not store any other way!). Take 1 teaspoon 3 times a day, one hour after meals. Do not overdose - this may have dangerous consequences. To achieve expected results, continue the therapy until the entire amount of juice from 22lb (10kg) is finished.

I would like to warn that people with lots of unhealthy deposits in the skeletal system might experience bone pain, sometimes quite intensive. Do not be afraid and do not take painkillers. Simply continue the therapy. This phenomenon is normal during the cleansing process. A successful therapy can free you from much pain in the future.

If you experience liver pain (this may happen when the gallbladder is cleansed of stones and salt), put an electric thermal pad on your liver for 40-60 minutes. If there are no liver pains, increase the amount to 2-3 teaspoons after 7 days. Avoid hot and sour foods during the therapy and limit the consumption of bread, fish, eggs, milk and dairy products. Eat more natural plant-based foods.

Do not discard the pulp from the radishes. Put it in a pot, add 10.6oz (300g) of honey, stir, cover with a lid, and put something heavy on top of it. Keep it in a dry, warm place and stir with a wooden spoon from time to time. When the juice is used up, you can start eating the pulp (it should be sour by then). Take 1-2 tablespoons with your meals. **Based on my patientsí testimonies, this therapy works like youth elixir - it makes them feel younger and more energetic. Wrinkles disappear and the complexion on their faces becomes fresh and healthy. Pains in the lower back, upper and lower limbs, muscles, etc. disappear completely.** I use this therapy every five years and people who see me only occasionally say that aging does not affect me.

Cleansing radionuclides and heavy metals from the body

Radionuclides and heavy metals are carcinogenic factors - they cause the development of cancer cells in our body. They get into our body with air, water, and food. All city dwellers without exception have high levels of these substances and are at risk of developing cancer in one of their organs. This is why cleansing the body of radionuclides and heavy metals should be an integral part of our hygiene.

Method A - using pine buds

Put 4 tablespoons of young pine buds into a half-quart (liter) jar, pour a cup of honey over it, and put it in the refrigerator. The buds will start producing juice after two days. Take 1 tablespoon of this juice 3 times a day.

Method B – using pine or spruce needles

Pour 1 quart (1L) of boiled water over 0.5 cup of cut-up pine or spruce needles, slowly warm up for 10-15 minutes almost to the point of boiling, then strain the brew. Drink 1-2 cups twice a day for seven days instead of tea, take a two-month interval, and repeat for another seven days. Use this therapy once a year.

Method C – using flax seed

Pour 1.5 quart (1.5L) of boiling water over 0.5 cup of flax seed, cook it for two hours on low heat, cool it off and strain. Drink it out throughout the day. Use the therapy once a year for two weeks.

Sucking oil

This method can be used in the treatment of vein inflammations, chronic anemia, paralysis, eczema, swelling, gastrointestinal disorders, heart and circulatory disorders, cancers, joint disorders, and many other health conditions, which may be less serious but still troublesome.

You have probably seen little children sucking on their thumbs. This reflex is provided by nature as part of the child's self-preservation instinct. Its task is to produce large amounts of saliva, which has an antibacterial effect.

This is probably where folk medicine got the idea for a therapy, which uses a similar mechanism – holding vegetable oil in the mouth for about 30 minutes produces a therapeutic effect.

The amount of blood circulated through our mouth area in 30 minutes equals 3.5-4 quarts (3.5-4L). Vegetable oil has good absorbing qualities. The therapeutic method described below uses these qualities to absorb toxic substances from our body.

The method is simple, painless, and absolutely harmless. Many generations of Siberian healers used it with good effects. The essential steps of the procedure are the following:

The therapy should be done on an empty stomach in the morning or before bedtime in the evening (3-4 hours after your last meal). Use not more than 1 tablespoon of sunflower oil or peanut oil, hold it in the front part of your mouth, and perform with your mouth, for 25-30 minutes, an action similar to sucking on a candy. The sucking action should not be very intense. The oil will thicken first and then it will become more liquid and white. Make sure you spit out the oil after the procedure. It should not be swallowed because it contains substances that cause many diseases. You can use the method as long as needed. Eventually you will feel refreshed, energetic, and calm. You will also regain good sleep and memory. Acute diseases are cured quickly – within 2-3 weeks. Chronic conditions take several months to a year and we should be aware that the therapy might trigger certain mild symptoms (e.g. the feeling of weakness) during the first week. This phenomenon is associated with the weakening of the disease's focal points. It is normal and we need to go through the experience. Properly implemented therapy will bring such noticeable signs as more energy on awakening, better appetite, and the feeling of freshness. Based on the state of your health, you can make your own decision about the duration of the therapy. Healthy people and children can use the method for two weeks as a preventative measure. This will not only prevent diseases mentioned above but also remove toxic heavy metals that can be found even in a healthy body. I do not need to convince anybody that prevention is better than treatment. The method brings best results if used daily for 1-6 months.

Dear Readers,

Now you can decide on your individual path towards good health. I perfectly realize that taking such step is not easy. In order to become healthy you have to quit bad habits formed over many years, change your lifestyle, and reform your way of thinking. If you feel that your health has begun deteriorating, waste no time – start acting quickly and take better care of yourself.

The sooner you start acting the speedier your health will be restored! It is important to make gradual lifestyle changes and allow your body enough time for adjustment.

This book is intended to be a practical health maintenance guide. If you use it frequently, you will surely find help in health matters. I encourage you to compare the information contained in this book with your own observations. Accumulate as much experience as possible and pass it on to your children and grandchildren. This will lead your entire family to good health for generations.

I hope you have found this book helpful. If you have any other questions, I invite you to explore the pages of my other books.

I wish you Good Health.

Mikhail Tombak

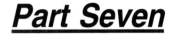

Part Seven

HEALTH WITHOUT MEDICATIONS

FOLK MEDICINE FORMULAS

Many letters from my readers repeat the same question: Is it safe for a diabetic to use remedies against high blood pressure, strong cough, or in fluenza?

All remedies described below contain only natural ingredients. This means that they can be used simultaneously without the risk of any harmful interaction or conflict. If we use four or five formulas at the same time, we should reduce their dosages by half.

A few remarks on preparing formulas:

➤ It is best to use enamel or glass vessels.
➤ Use wooden spoons for stirring ingredients.
➤ Store the jars with formulas on the lowest refrigerator shelf if possible.
➤ It is a good idea to use labels containing the recipe number, preparation date, ingredients, etc.
➤ Even though most formulas can be safely stored for a relatively long time,
I would recommend a maximum storage time of 6 months

Weather-related diseases

Treating sore throat, flu, coughing, runny nose, bronchitis

1. **Ingredients:** 1 tablespoon of raspberry jam, 1 tablespoon of honey, 1 tablespoon of vodka or brandy, 0.5 lemon
Preparation: Put all ingredients in a cup (250ml), squeeze the juice from the lemon, and add boiling water to fill the cup.
Usage: Drink 3 teaspoons in small sips before going to bed.

2. **Ingredients:** Juice squeezed from 1 lemon, 3.5oz (100g) of honey
Preparation: Mix the lemon juice with honey.
Usage: Take 1 tablespoon 3 times a day.

3. **Ingredients:** 3.5oz (100g) of lime flowers, 3.5oz (100g) of dried raspberries, 1 quart (1L) of boiling water

Preparation: Pour boiling water over the lime flowers and raspberries; let it stand for 10-15 minutes and strain the brew. **Usage:** Drink 7oz (200g) of warm brew before bedtime for 2-3 days. Store refrigerated and warm up before use.

4. **Ingredients:** 0.5 cup of radish juice 0.5 cup of grated horseradish, 0.5 cup of honey
   Preparation: Mix well and let stand for 3-4 hours.
   Usage: Take 3 times a day, 2-3 tablespoons for adults and 1 teaspoon for children. Store refrigerated.

5. **Ingredients:** 1.8oz (50g) of grated onion, 0.7oz (20g) of apple cider vinegar or wine vinegar, 2.1oz (60g) of honey
   Preparation: Pour vinegar over the onion. Add honey, mix everything together, let stand for 2 hours, and strain.
   Usage: Take 1 teaspoon every half an hour.

6. **Ingredients:** 3.5oz (100g) of grated onion, 3.5oz (100g) of sugar crystals
   Preparation: Put sugar on top of the onion and let stand for 1 hour. Store refrigerated.
   Usage: Take 2 teaspoons of juice secreted from the onion 3 times a day.

7. **Ingredients**: 3.5oz (100g) of garlic, 3.5oz (100g) of honey
   Preparation: Squeeze juice from the garlic, mix with honey, let stand for 24 hours and strain into a 7 fl oz (200ml) jar. Store refrigerated.
   Usage: Take 1 teaspoon 3 times a day or 1 tablespoon before bedtime. Drink some warm water with it.

Treating sore throat, colds, and coughing

8. **Ingredients:** 0.5 cup of milk, 4 or 5 figs
   Preparation: Put together in a pot, cook for 5-10 minutes, and let it cool off.
   Usage: Drink the milk in small sips and eat the figs before bedtime. Repeat the therapy 3-4 times if coughing persists.

Treating colds and coughing

9. **Ingredients:** 0.5 cup of honey 0.5 cup of red dry wine, 0.35-0.53oz (10-15g) of garlic
   Preparation: Pour the wine over the honey and mix well. Peel and crush the garlic.
   Usage: Rub the crushed garlic on your feet before going to bed and put on woolen socks. Put on warm pajamas, warm up the wine and drink it.

Remedies against coughing

10. **Ingredients:** 7oz (200g) of unsalted butter, 7oz (200g) of lard, 7oz (200g) of honey, 7oz (200g) of cocoa powder, 15 egg yolks
    Preparation: Mix everything together; heat up to the point of boiling and cook slowly for 30-40 minutes, and let it cool off. Store refrigerated.
    Usage: Take 1 teaspoon with 1/2 cup of hot milk 3 times a day. Drink in small sips. It should bring results in 5-7 days.

11. **Ingredients:** 2 tablespoons of hot boiled milk, 2 tablespoons of brandy
    Preparation: Mix ingredients together.
    Usage: Take half an hour before meals 3 times a day. Do not spend time in cool weather immediately after – do not let your body cool off. Take until cured

12. **Ingredients:** 0.33 quart (0.33L) of beer and 1 tablespoon of honey
    Preparation: Put together in an enamel pot, cook slowly for 5 minutes.
    Usage: Drink warm in small sips 2 times a week.

Remedy against occasional heavy and night coughing

13. **Ingredients:** 1 lemon, 2 tablespoons of glycerin, some honey
    Preparation: Cook the lemon slowly for 10 minutes (it will become softer and yield more juice). Cut it in half, squeeze

217

into jar (about 1 Cup / 200-250 ml), add glycerin, mix well, and add honey to fill the jar. Close tightly.

Usage: Take 1 teaspoon before bedtime and 1 more at night in case of night coughing. Keep refrigerated.

Cough remedy for elderly people

14. Ingredients: 7oz (200g) of butter, 7oz (200g) of lard, 7oz (200g) of honey

Preparation: Mix in a pot, cook slowly for five minutes (until it becomes a uniform pulp), and let it cool off.

Usage: Mix 1 teaspoon with 0.5 cup of hot milk and drink in small sips 3 times a day 1 - 1.5 hour after meals.

Treating sore throat

15. Ingredients: 1 cup of grated red beet and 1 cup of apple cider vinegar or wine vinegar

Preparation: Pour the vinegar over the beet, let it stand for 2-3 hours, and strain into a glass vessel.

Usage: Rinse your throat and drink 1 tablespoon twice a day.

In case of flu outbreak

Onions and garlic occupy the top positions in all folk flu prevention formulas.

They are to be eaten or at least chewed for 2-3 minutes, preferably before bedtime.

You can use the following garlic formula for prevention during flu outbreaks:

16. Ingredients: 2 or 3 garlic cloves, 1-1.7 fl oz (30-50ml) of boiling water.

Preparation: Chop the garlic finely, pour boiling water over it, and let it stand 1-2 hours, and strain (store for up to 2 days, keep refrigerated).

Usage: Use as nose drops 1 or 2 times a day - 2 or 3 drops into each nostril.

> ➤ To avoid infecting your family, you can hang a small cotton bag with finely chopped garlic on your neck (2 or 3 cloves). To protect small children from the outbreak, put such cotton bag or a small plate with chopped garlic next to their beds.

> ➤ Another way of flu prevention is chewing a eucalyptus leaf every morning and keeping a piece of such leaf in your mouth (between the gum and the cheek) during contacts with flu-infected people. You can also rinse your throat every evening with freshly squeezed raw beet juice blended with a teaspoon of 3% vinegar.

Use the following advice if you cannot prevent the infection and become ill.

> ➤ Drink hot tea with lemon (or raspberry jam) or warm milk with honey (1 tablespoon per cup) as often as possible.
> ➤ Put cotton swabs dipped in fresh onion juice into your nostrils for seven minutes 3-4 times a day.
> ➤ Squeeze an onion into a little bowl and sniff the juice for 2-3 minutes 3 times a day.
> ➤ Grate finely a head of garlic and mix with an equal amount of honey (lime honey is best). Take 1 tablespoon before bedtime and drink some warm water.
> ➤ Grate an onion, pour 0.5 quart (0.5L) of boiling milk over it and store in a warm place. Drink hot - half of it before bedtime and half in the morning.
> ➤ Pour 1 cup of boiling water over 2 tablespoons of dried (or 3.5oz/100g of fresh) raspberries. Let it stand for 10-15 minutes, add 1 tablespoon of honey, and mix well. Take warm before bedtime to stimulate sweating.

Treating hoarseness

Folk medicine formulas are recommended in cases of sore throat following a cold. They are not as suitable as remedies against acute throat inflammations.

> Wash a pear, peel it, and squeeze juice from it. Drink it in small sips from time to time, holding each sip in your mouth for a while.
> Wash a few olives and hold them in your mouth for a while one by one while swallowing your saliva.
> Eat 5-10 chunks of white turnip 3 times a day.

Digestive system disorders

Stomach ulceration, stomach bleeds

17. **Ingredients:** 4 tablespoons (20g) of fine dry oak bark, 1 cup of boiling water
Preparation: Put the bark in an enamel pot, pour boiling water over it, cover it with a lid, and boil for 20 minutes stirring from time to time. Let it cool off, strain, pour it in a tightly closed glass container in a dark place, and store in a dark place.
Usage: Take 1 tablespoon 2-3 times a day.

Liver disorders

Stimulating the secretion of bile in cases of liver disorders

18. **Ingredients:** 3.5oz (100g) of wild rose fruits, some sugar
Preparation: Put the wild rose fruit in a one-liter thermos, fill the thermos with boiling water, close it, and let it stand overnight.
Usage: Drink the entire brew over 1 day adding some sugar for better taste.

Treating gallstones

19. **Ingredients:** A handful of dried birch leaves
Preparation: Break up the leaves, pour 1 cup of boiling water over them, let the brew stand for 20 minutes (stir with a wooden spoon from time to time), and strain it.

Usage: Take 1 cup of the brew before meals in the morning and the evening.

20. Ingredients: A black radish
Preparation: Grate the black radish and squeeze juice from it.
Usage: Take 2-3 tablespoons of fresh juice every day.

Liver colic, liver stones

21. Ingredients: 10 dried figs, 1 cup of boiling water, 0.5 cup of hot milk, and 1 teaspoon of sugar
Preparation: Chop the figs finely, put them in an enamel pot, pour boiling water over them, bring to the point of boiling, add milk and sugar, and let it cool off.
Usage: Drink the liquid in small sips while still warm and eat the figs.

Treating hemorrhoids, liver disorders, or constipation

22. Ingredients: Sauerkraut juice
Usage: Drink 0.5 -1 cup of juice a day an hour before a meal for 14-30 days.

Kidney and bladder disorders

Stimulating urination and treating kidney and bladder stones

23. Ingredients: Juice squeezed from a horseradish (both root and leaves)
Usage: Take 1 teaspoon of freshly squeezed juice every morning and evening.

24. Ingredients: 1 teaspoon of tea extract and 1.7oz (50g) of sage.
Preparation: Put the ingredients in a one-liter thermos, pour boiling water over them, and let them stand for 30 minutes.
Usage: Drink half a cup 6-8 times a day.

25. **Ingredients:** 1 cup of honey and 1 cup of sauerkraut juice
Preparation: Mix together, pour in a glass bottle, close the bottle, and store in a cool dark place.
Usage: Take 1 tablespoon 3 times a day one hour before meals.

26. **Ingredients:** 3.5oz (100g) of unripe green walnuts (harvested before Jul 7) and 3.5oz (100g) of sugar crystals or honey
Preparation: Chop the walnuts finely, put them in a jar, add sugar or honey, close the jar tightly, and keep in the refrigerator for 1 month.
Usage: Take 1 teaspoon 3 times a day before meals. Store refrigerated.

Treating kidney stones, liver stones, and gallstones

27. **Ingredients:** 3 lemons (with peel but without seeds, 5.3oz (150g) of peeled garlic, 0.5 quart (0.5L) of cool boiled water
Preparation: Grind lemon together with garlic, put in a 1 quart (1L) jar, fill the jar with water, let it stand 24 hours, strain it, close the jar tightly, and store in a dark place.
Usage: Drink 1.7 fl oz (50 ml) every morning.

28. **Ingredients:** 3 cups of water, 4 lemons (without seeds), 1 cup of honey, and juice from 1 lemon
Preparation: Pour the water into a pot and add finely chopped lemons. Boil until there is only about 1 cup of brew left, let it cool off, strain it, pour in a glass container, add honey and lemon juice, mix well, and cover with a lid.
Usage: Take 1 tablespoon every day before bedtime until finished. Store refrigerated.

In case of kidney colic, put an electric heating pad on your kidney area or take a hot bath.
Caution: Acute inflammations of other abdominal organs may cause similar pains. If you are not sure that the pain is caused by kidney colic, do not follow the advice given above and contact a physician.

Treating kidney sand

29. Ingredients: 1 lemon (without seeds), 1.8oz (50g) of honey, 1.8oz (50g) of vegetable oil
Preparation: Put the lemon into boiling water for a moment, then dry it, grate, put in a glass container, add honey and oil, mix everything well, and cover with a lid.
Usage: Take 1 tablespoon 4-5 times a day.

Cardiovascular disorders

In case of cardiovascular disorders:

➢ Take 1 teaspoon of honey with milk or whole cottage cheese 2-3 times a day.
➢ Drink a cup of warm tea with a tablespoon of honey every day before bedtime.

30. Ingredients: 7oz (200g) of raisins, 1 quart (1L) of boiling water, 1 tablespoon of fresh lemon juice
Preparation: Wash the raisins, pour boiling water on them and boil for another 5 minutes. Let it cool off, strain, add lemon juice, and close tightly in a glass container.
Usage: Take 0.5 cup 3 times a day for 1-2 months. Store refrigerated.

31. Ingredients: 1 tablespoon of carrot juice, 1e tablespoon of grated horseradish, 1 cup of honey, juice from 1 lemon
Preparation: Mix well with a wooden spoon in an enamel pot, put in a glass container, close tightly, and store in a cool place.
Usage: Take 1 teaspoon 3 times a day (one hour before meals) for 2 months.

Reducing blood pressure in case of weak heart function

32. **Ingredients:** 1 tablespoon of melissa leaves, 1 cup of boiling water
    Preparation: Pour boiling water over melissa leaves, let it stand for 1 hour, and strain the brew.
    Usage: Take 1 tablespoon 3 times a day.

To strengthen a weakened heart

Chew on a piece of lemon peel every day – it is rich in ethereal oils.

High blood pressure

To reduce blood pressure, it is necessary to cleanse the circulatory system and the liver (see Complete Body Cleansing — part six). Limit you intake of fats and flour-based products. Eat more foods rich in vitamin C and be more physically active.

33. **Ingredients:** 0.5 quart (0.5L) of vodka and 7oz (200g) of chopped garlic
    Preparation: Pour vodka into a 0.75 quart (0.75L) dark glass bottle, add garlic, close tight, and let it stand in a dark place for 6-8 days (shake it from time to time). Strain the formula, close tightly, and store refrigerated.
    Usage: Take 1 tablespoon 3 times a day before meals.

High blood pressure, heart disorders, disseminated encephalomyelitis

34. **Ingredients:** 1 lemon without seeds, 7oz (200g) of cranberry, 7oz (200g) of wild rose fruit, 7oz (200g) of honey
    Preparation: Put the lemon into boiling water for a while, dry it with a piece of cloth, and grate finely. Crush the cranberry and wild rose fruits. Put everything in a glass container, add honey, mix well, and let it stand for 24 hours.

Usage: Take 1 tablespoon 3 times a day 15 minutes before meals for 14-30 days.

Low blood pressure

People with a tendency to low blood pressure should be physically active – walk and run as much as possible.

➢ Take 1 teaspoon of honey with milk or whole cottage cheese 2-3 times a day.
➢ Regular use of sauna once a week for a year normalizes blood pressure.
➢ Alternate hot and cold showers wonderfully regulate the tone of blood vessels.
➢ Vibration massage helps increase blood pressure: Stand straight on your toes, your arms along your body, and then forcefully drop your body weight on your heels. Repeat 20 times in the morning and the evening. An alternate rhythmic stumping of your heels against the floor increases your blood pressure.
➢ If your blood pressure decreases during weather changes, drink at least 1 cup of carrot juice (four parts) mixed with beet juice (one part).

Treating arteriosclerosis

➢ Drink half a cup of juice squeezed from raw potatoes on an empty stomach in the morning for 14 days.
➢ Take a lemon therapy.
➢ Cleanse your liver.
➢ Eat 1 grapefruit on an empty stomach in the morning and 1 in the evening two hours after your last meal.
➢ Drink 2-3 cups of green tea every day.
➢ Cleanse your lymphatic system.
➢ Take alternate hot and cold showers in the morning and the afternoon.

> Drink 1/3 cup of pumpkin juice, a cup of watermelon juice, or 1/3 cup of beet juice 3 times a day, 15 minutes before meals.
> Mix juice from half a grapefruit and mix it with 1 tablespoon of olive oil. Take everyday for one month and make one-month interval before repeating. Use this therapy once a year.
> Grind and mix walnuts, raisins, honey, and figs - 3.5oz (100g) each. Take 1 tablespoon or as a spread twice a day.
> Squeeze juice from 1.7oz (50g) of garlic, add a cup of vodka to it, and let it stand in a warm place for 3 days. Take 8 drops followed by a gulp of cold water 3 times a day.

35. **Ingredients:** Juice from 2 large heads of garlic and 8.8oz (250g) of vodka
Preparation: Pour vodka on top of garlic juice in a half-liter jar and let it stand in a dark place for 12 days.
Usage: Take 20 drops 3 times a day (30 minutes before meals) for 3 weeks. Take a month interval; repeat for another 3 weeks, and so on until the supply is finished.

Pains in joints, bones, and muscles

36. **Ingredients:** 1.5 cup of black radish juice, 1 cup of honey, 5 fl oz (150ml) of vodka (40% proof or up), 1 tablespoon of salt
Preparation: Mix everything together.
Usage: Take 1 tablespoon before bedtime, store refrigerated.

37. **Ingredients:** 0.5 quart (0.5L) of vodka (40% proof or up), 5 pods of hot pepper 2.5-3 inches (6-8cm) long.
Preparation: Chop the pepper pods finely, put in a jar, pour spirit over it cover with a lid, and let it stand in a dark place for a week.
Usage: Soak a piece of cotton cloth in the formula on cover the affected area for 3-4 hours. Even the most persistent pains should disappear after 7-10 sessions.
You can also rub the formula on your aching joints and muscles (once a day before bedtime). This usually removes pain after 12-15 days.

38. Ingredients: 1.8oz (50g) of camphor, 1.8oz (50g) of powdered mustard seed, 0.35oz (10g) of vodka (40% proof or up), 3.5oz (100g) of raw egg white.
Preparation: Pour spirit in a jar, add camphor, and let it dissolve. Add and dissolve mustard seed powder, add egg white, and stir to form a thick pulp. Keep refrigerated and warm up slightly before each use.
Usage: Rub on the effected muscle and joint areas before bedtime. Do not rub in completely – let it leave a film on your skin for 20 minutes and then wash the excess off with a piece of cotton cloth soaked in warm water.

Diabetes

39. Ingredients: 3.5oz (100g) of onion juice and 3.5oz (100g) of honey
Preparation: Peel 1 onion, grate it finely, squeeze the juice into a jar, add honey, mix well, close tightly, and store in a dark place.
Usage: Take 2 teaspoons 3 times a day before meals for one month.

40. Ingredients: 10 average-sized bay leaves, about 2 cups (0.5L) of boiling water
Preparation: Break up the leaves, put in a half-liter thermos, pour boiling water over them, and let it stand for 2-3 hours.
Usage: Drink half a cup of warm formula 3-4 times a day before meals for two weeks.

Menopause

To delay menopause, use the following therapy starting at the age of forty:

41. Ingredients: 7oz (200g) of white wine and 10-12 cloves of garlic.

Preparation: Slowly heat up wine to the point of boiling, add garlic and boil for another 30 seconds, let it cool off and pour in a dark glass bottle. Store in a dark place at room temperature.

Usage: Take 1 tablespoon 3 times a day 20 minutes before meals for 3 days in a row (day 1, 2, 3; 11, 12, 13; 21, 22, 23 of each month). The therapy also brings back the childbearing ability, improves skin complexion, and brings the sense of wellbeing.

Formula used to stop bleeding and eliminate unpleasant symptoms of menopause

42. **Ingredients:** Peel from ten oranges, 2 quarts (2L) of boiling water, some sugar or honey

    Preparation: Put orange peels in boiling water, cover the pot with a lid, and boil slowly until there is only about 0.7 quart (0.7L) of fluid left. Strain the brew twice and add sugar or honey for better taste. Pour the formula in a bottle and store refrigerated.

    Usage: Take 1 tablespoon 3-4 times a day

Eyes

➢ Pour 0.5 a cup of boiling water over 0.5 a cup of cucumber peels and add 0.5 a teaspoon of baking soda. Use for compresses.

➢ Cook an onion (with peel) in a small amount of water, add some honey to the brew and mix well. Rinse your eyes with the brew 4-5 times a day (it removes the redness).

➢ Grate an apple or potato, mix it with an egg white, and put on the eyes. Rinse off with warm boiled water.

Burns

➢ Put finely grated carrot on the affected area.

➢ Mix an egg yolk with a teaspoon of butter (it should resemble mayonnaise), put on a soft pad and apply on the affected area. It will relieve pain and prevent scars.

➤ Rinse the affected area under cold water and generously apply baking soda.

➤ In case of burns in the throat, rinse it with 1 tablespoon of oil and swallow the oil.

Dropsy

➤ Vegetables and fruits that have diuretic qualities are recommended – celery, parsnips, asparagus, onion, garlic, watermelon, wild strawberries, and currants.

43. Ingredients: 2 average-sized onions and 1 tablespoon of sugar
Preparation: Slice the onions in the evening, put sugar on top, let it stand overnight (the onion should start secreting juice), squeeze juice from the onions in the morning.
Usage: Take 2 tablespoons a day.

➤ Drink 0.5 a cup of pumpkin juice a day.

Rejuvenating the body after a serious illness

Body-strengthening formula

44. Ingredients: Nuts, apricots, raisins, dried plums, sunflower seeds, and honey – 3.5oz (100g) each, 2 lemons with peel (without seeds)
Preparation: Grind everything, add honey, mix well, and store in a closed 1 quart (1L) glass container in a cool place.
Usage: Take 2-4 teaspoons during a day (adults). Use 1 teaspoon a day for children.

Healing power of apple cider vinegar

Apple cider vinegar

Many people use large amounts of vinegar for seasoning or in preparation of food products. Wine vinegar and white distilled vinegar contain ingredients that harm our health, for example acetic acid ($C_2H_4O_2$). Acetic acid destroys red blood cells, causes anemia, interferes with the digestive processes, and impedes food absorption. It causes cirrhosis (a chronic liver disease), ulcerative inflammations of the large intestine, etc. (beware if you like pickled cucumbers and mushrooms or different pickled salads). My advice is not to use spirit vinegar to avoid digestive tract problems.

Apple cider vinegar has entirely different qualities. It contains malic acid ($C_4H_6O_5$). When it reacts with bases and minerals, it produces glycogen, which helps regulate the menstrual cycle, improves the condition of blood vessels, and promotes the building of red blood cells. One of the most valuable qualities of apple vinegar is very high content of potassium, necessary for calming the nervous system, regulating the hormonal function, and retaining calcium, iron, magnesium, and silicon in our body.

Apple vinegar can be bought in stores or prepared at home.

Making apple cider vinegar

The amount of ingredients depending on the amount of apple cider vinegar you need for your specific use. Cut out rotten and damaged parts of the apples. Grind or crush the apples (including the peel and seeds with their enclosures). Put the pulp in an enamel or glass container with a wide opening and add warm boiled water (1 quart/1L of water per 28oz/800g of apple pulp). Add 3.5oz (100g) of honey, 0.35oz (10g) of baker's yeast, and 0.7oz (20g) of dried dark bread per 1 quart (1L) of water. Cover the container with a lid and let it stand in the temperature of 68-86F (20-30C) for fermentation (steady temperature and wide container opening improve fermentation). Stir it with a wooden spoon every day. After ten days, put it in a gauze bag and squeeze juice from it. Filter the juice into a container with a wide opening. Add 2.8oz (80g) of honey per 1 quart (1L) of juice and stir until honey is dissolved. Cover the container with a gauze pad and let it stand in the temperature of 77-86F (25-30C). The vinegar is ready when its color turns light. It usually takes 40-60 days, depending on the kind of apples, honey, the amount of water, and some other factors. When the fluid turns light, use a funnel to pour it into half-liter bottles, close the bottles tightly with a cork stopper (you can pour some wax on top of the stopper to close it more tightly), and store in a cool place. You can use it as a remedy (see the section below) or as seasoning with your salads and other food. I would like to stress again, that apple cider vinegar is the only acidic seasoning to be used with your food.

Apple cider vinegar therapies

Limping caused by an injury

Mix 1 egg yolk with 1 teaspoon of honey, and 1 teaspoon of apple cider vinegar. Rub the mixture on the affected area.

Shingles

Apply a gauze pad soaked in undiluted apple cider vinegar on the affected areas 4 times during the day and 3 times at night (if itching does not let you sleep). The remedy relieves the pain in 5-10 minutes and cures shingles in 3-7 days.

Night sweating

Rub apple vinegar on your skin before bedtime.

Burns

Use a gauze pad soaked in apple cider vinegar to wash the affected areas. It relieves pain and prevents scarring.

Varicose veins

Wash the skin in the area of dilated veins with a pad soaked in apple cider vinegar in the morning and the evening. In addition, drink a solution of 2 teaspoons of apple cider vinegar in a cup of warm boiled water 2 times a day. The dilated veins usually start narrowing after a month of regular therapy.

Weight reduction therapy

Drink a cup of boiled water with 2 teaspoons of apple cider vinegar before every meal.

Excessive secretion of tears

Make a solution of 1 teaspoon of apple cider vinegar and 1 drop of iodine in 1 cup of water. Drink every day for 2 weeks; then drink twice a week (e.g. Tuesday and Thursday) for two months.

Limping caused by joint inflammation

Take 10 teaspoons of apple cider vinegar before every meal. The therapy should reduce pain in 20% after 2 days, 50% after 5 days, and remove the pain completely after 30 days.

High blood pressure

Some people have high blood pressure caused by a deficiency of hydrochloric acid in their digestive tract. It is necessary to lower the intake of meat to effectively treat this condition. A noticeable reduction of blood pressure can be achieved by taking 1 to 3 teaspoons of apple cider vinegar before every meal. For better effects, you can occasionally take apple cider vinegar with a teaspoon of honey,

Headaches

Pour half a cup of apple cider vinegar and half a cup of boiled water in a pot. Mix the solution, heat up slowly to the point of boiling, and turn off the heat. Slowly inhale the vapor 75 times. The headache will be removed or at least significantly reduced.

APPENDIX A

Interviews with the Author

In Harmony with Nature
An interview with "Express Ilustrowany"

Is it not true that we have an arsenal of sophisticated medications against all diseases?
   We indeed do. However, we forgot the simple truth that pain is a signal from our body that something is going wrong. When we started looking for means to remove pain, we invented medications, which do not remove the causes of the problem, just its symptoms. Increased number of drugs caused an increased number of diseases because all drugs have side-effects and, while fighting one disease, create another one. This caused a multitude of problems affecting all bodily organs and, for the sake of convenience, medicine became specialized in treating particular component parts of the human body. This way an integral and complex system, described as body and soul became divided into the heart, kidneys, liver, nervous system, brain, spinal cord, etc. Cardiologists started treating the heart, urologists – kidneys, laryngologists – ears, throat and nose. From that moment on, we no longer existed as a whole. Despite powerful drugs and perfected medical technology, we are still subjected to disease. Hundreds of thousands die from cancer every year, millions die from heart attacks and, what is particularly interesting, richer societies suffer from more serious and complicated diseases. This happens because nobody can produce medication against the habits of overeating, improper breathing, and physical inactivity – that is, against unhealthy lifestyle.

Have we seen the worst?
   Unfortunately we have not. What causes concern among scientists and doctors all over the world is the fact that most people's immune system is already weakened at the age of twenty. Even the strongest antibiotics are ineffective against some new viral infections. Germs

233

declared a war on humans and its outcome is unpredictable. Weakened immune system is an effect of violating the laws of nature.

You maintain that damage to our health starts as early as in our infancy.

The only food appropriate for infants is mother's milk – nature itself provides it. Only mother's milk creates healthy microflora in the large intestine with bacteria that protect the infant against all infections. Milk contributes to the development of the natural self-preservation instinct. However, if an infant is fed artificial food practically from the time of birth, the large intestine degenerates and is not able to protect the child against diseases. The body has low immunity and frequently becomes ill. In order to fight diseases, we stuff our children with antibiotics that destroy all microorganisms, both disease-causing and friendly. This causes frequent constipation – a problem that becomes even more aggravated by high consumption of refined and synthetic products. As a result, the body suffers from a condition called disbacteriosis, which means the degeneration of healthy microflora and a damaged immune system. Can we expect such a child to be healthy?

Why are more and more dangerous disease-causing bacteria developing in our body?

As we know, disease-causing bacteria best develop in alkaline environment. Excessive consumption of meat, sweets, and white baked goods promotes alkaline environment in our body. If we use incorrect diet for many years, we create ideal conditions for the development of unfriendly bacteria.

It takes many years to implement a newly invented antibiotic and the bacteria it was designed against have enough time to modify. Nature does not invent new medications. Garlic has been used for many hundreds of years against all kinds of infections and it will remain the best antibiotic.

There is no perfect medication effective against all diseases, is there?

I do not believe commercials that offer unusually effective remedies against all diseases. There are no miracle drugs. Neither are there any easy methods to maintain good health. We cannot buy health in a pharmacy.

What advice would you offer our readers who desire to live long and be healthy?

Return to simple natural diet, learn to breathe correctly, use a lot of physical exercise, and expose your body to water, air, and sunlight. When we live in harmony with nature, our body heals and rejuvenates by itself.

***

Fragments of an interview with Professor Mikhail Tombak conducted by Bohdan Gadomski of ANGORA weekly.

BOHDAN GADOMSKI, the host of this interview, is one of the most popular press publicists in Poland. He is also well known in Polish emigration circles in the USA, Canada, and Europe as the editor of "Angora" weekly where, in the column "Bohdan Gadomski's Salon Storms" he publicizes his interviews with the most interesting personalities of Polish cultural and social scene. His record includes several thousand interviews, some of them well publicized and widely commented on. He can be considered a multimedia journalist because he also publicizes on the radio and television. He is currently working on the publication of an anthology of his most famous interviews, "Under the Beds of Stars."

Your advice on ways of attaining a long and healthy life started a lot of controversy. I would like to know where and how you gained knowledge that you recently started sharing with other people.

During my university years, I took part in a scientific expedition to the Far East where I met with Tibetan monks. Their approach to the human body is different and very interesting. I learned some secrets from them that allow diagnosing disorders from the way people look, walk, or even wear out their shoes. I also became convinced that it is never just a single organ that is ill in a human body. When something causes us pain and we start treating it, we are fighting symptoms and do not address causes. This is why the problem can manifest itself in some other place, causing pain associated with a completely different disease. I do not treat diseases as something concrete. They are just irregularities in our body's normal functioning.

Why did you choose biology and not medicine as your area of study?

I come from a medical family. As a child, I asked my mother why she was not able to cure my ill father and why she was suffering from heartaches and insomnia. When I did not get an answer, I understood that medicine concerns itself only with the application of drugs. Biology is a much more comprehensive science that allows inquiring about every little detail of human body. This is why I chose biology, even though my mother wished me to study medicine.

According to your writings, "health depends not only on correct diet, but also ..."

It also depends on correct breathing. We can survive a month without food, but hardly a few minutes without air. We cannot be healthy as long as we breathe incorrectly. Nine people out of ten breathe improperly, causing chronic oxygen deficiency in their body. This causes them to age prematurely and to suffer from all kinds of diseases.

What causes most damage to our health?

There are several factors: incorrect breathing, improper eating and drinking, not enough exercise and joy of life, and also such emotions as envy, greed, or anger. We constantly have problems and dilemmas and this significantly shortens our life.

You wrote that people are like trees. Where is the resemblance?

We have a supporting structure in the form of our spine. We have roots that nurture us. If anything goes wrong with the spine, we become prone to various diseases.

Can aging be delayed?

Our life could be very long if we did not shorten it ourselves. I once met two old men in Georgia (Caucasus), one was 160 years old and the other 120 years old. They were both slim and still enjoyed dance and singing. They only ate freshly prepared food – all their meals were prepared shortly before they were eaten. They were both constantly on the move, kept smiling, and had generally a very positive attitude towards life. In reality, humans do not have to age. Old Testament patriarchs lived up to 950 years. Our kidneys, according to a

236

scientifically designed model, could last 1200 years. However, we cause our kidneys to be stuffed with stones by the age of 35 and when we are over 50, our health becomes generally weak and we spend most of our time fighting health problems.

You promote a healthy lifestyle. Have you always been healthy yourself?

I had once liver cirrhosis, caused by improper nutrition administered by my mother-physician. During my childhood, I frequently suffered from constipation. Spinal injuries caused me to lose sensation in my lower limbs for two years. According to doctors, I had no chance to walk again.

Who is better off: meat-eaters or vegetarians?

According to statistics, vegetarians have higher endurance than meat-eaters, but both suffer from various diseases. It is best to use moderation in everything. It is one of the fundamental conditions of our survival. The only thing that should not be subject to moderation is smiling – the more the better.

There is huge interest in your work. Crowds of people used to camp in front of your house in Moscow day and night. You draw crowds in Poland as soon as you show up at the Festival of the Unusual. Why do you refuse to see patients?

I do not see patients in Poland because this was the purpose of leaving Russia, where it was difficult for me to enter my own home. This kind of life became unbearable. Everything I know is contained in my books.

APPENDIX B

Excerpts from the Articles in the Monthly Magazine "Człowiek, Zdrowie, Natura –Szaman"

Nina Grella is a well-known Polish journalist and, for many years, a promoter of natural healing methods. Among her books is the bestseller "Natural Healing" and "I Can See without Glasses." She is the editor of "Czlowiek, Zdrowie, Natura – Szaman" monthly magazine and the organizer of the largest event promoting natural healing methods in Europe – the fair "Closer to Health, Closer to Nature."

Excerpts from the article "Mikhail Tombak's Health University" by Nina Grella in "Czlowiek, Zdrowie, Natura – Szaman" monthly magazine

From the moment in my life, when I met Professor Mikhail Tombak – (the event I consider one of the most significant facts in my professional life) – I've been trying to convince all my readers and listeners about the benefits of internal body cleansing. When we organized together the first therapeutic retreat for internal cleansing (it was described then as liver cleansing retreat), I already knew that the procedure not only alleviates liver problems but it also improves the functioning of other organs. I did not know, however, that it also clears human mind in an unusual way.

Excerpts from the article "The Week of Kindness for Body and Mind" by Nina Grella

Joanna
Just like a year ago, I am again at my computer to share everything I experienced and learned during two therapeutic liver-cleansing retreats

with Professor Mikhail Tombak. Last year's article was titled, "The Week of Kindness towards the Liver." This year I got finally convinced that it was not a week of kindness for only one organ. The effects of Professor Tombak's unusual therapy reach much deeper. They strengthen and heal the entire body and at the same time they change the patient's psychological condition. Joanna helped me realize this right after my arrival at Szczyrk. I noticed a somewhat familiar smiling face by the reception desk.

"Don't you recognize me?" – the blonde asked.

"I think I do but somehow it is hard for me to recall how we met." – I answered sincerely.

"I took part in last year's retreat with the Professor. You can certainly recall the asthmatic female that was not able to climb a flight of stairs without pausing and using the respirator."

"Is this you?" – I exclaimed – "I can't believe my own eyes! You look ten years younger."

"That's what everybody tells me; I simply lost ten kilos and, most important, got rid of my asthma."

"I felt wonderful after my return from Szczyrk." – she continued her story – "The constant sensation of air shortage disappeared and the fear of attacks was slowly diminishing. I realized two weeks later that I wasn't actually using my respirator anymore but I was still regularly taking medication prescribed by doctors. However, the decision to completely give up medication started maturing in my mind during the next days. I dared to take that step exactly one month after my return from the therapeutic retreat. I was terribly afraid but managed to stick to my decision all day. The next day fear wasn't there anymore. I took all medications out of my purse and ostentatiously left them on the table. While at work, I did not have anything for protection against asthma attacks. There was an overwhelming conviction that I was healthy and this conviction lasts till today. I became a totally different person during this year. I'm no longer a fearful person that constantly tries to hide behind somebody else's back. Instead, I have an extraordinary drive to be active and constantly come up with new ideas. My joyfulness and optimism amazes co-workers, friends, and family."

Barbara
Barbara was another person out of the group who came back to Szczyrk for a second time to perform the liver cleansing routine under the

Professor's supervision, listen to his fascinating lectures, and undergo a biotherapeutic spine alignment procedure, which indeed works miracles.

"I noticed that it removes cramps in muscles and tendons, stops acute migraine pains, straightens body posture, and is an excellent preparation for the liver-cleansing procedure.

This time I brought my twenty-year old son with me. When he saw the change in the state of my health after my return from the first retreat, he made his decision, without any need of my persuading, to undergo internal cleansing procedures. Wojtek has athletic ambitions and shows pretty good results. Unfortunately, he inherited from me a predisposition for allergies, which makes it hard for him to use his full potential. When he found out that I was able to set medication aside and regain an excellent physical condition along with good psychological disposition, he said one day, "I'm going as well."

Thanks to taking part in the retreat, listening to Professor's lectures, and attentive reading of his books, Barbara is regarded to be an expert on natural medicine in her circle of friends. She is convinced that performing lemon therapy and following other advice of the Professor saved the life of one of her friends' husband, who had a surgery done on his fourth-stage lung cancer.

Alicja

I noticed Alicja at the moment when her file was started by Dr. Hanna Chmiel-Pietriczenko, who took care of both groups of participants this year. I had known Alicja for many years and had reasons to believe that, once she decided to go through the liver-cleansing procedure, she would perform everything in a flawless manner. Since she lived in Katowice I knew, I would have the opportunity to follow the changes in the condition of her health, which was not vibrant.

"I decided to come to Szczyrk" – she said – "mainly because I felt terrible. I am 44lb (20 kg) overweight, my blood pressure is high (160/100), and constantly high heartbeat (100 per minute). My total cholesterol level is reaching 300mg/dL. In addition, I have been suffering frequent constipation since my youngest years. Bloating, pains in the right abdomen, and aching knees take a toll on me. Pain in my hands is so acute that I'm afraid I soon won't be able to hold a pen. I tried to get help from my family doctor first. Misdiagnosis and ineffective treatment forced me to try other clinics. I got some immediate relief but I feel that they were just treating the worst symptoms of some undiagnosed disease. I decided to take matters in my own hands and here I am."

Alicja is the kind of patient that doctors describe as difficult. She wants to know and understand everything about the treatment. Skepticism is an integral part of her mentality and it shows at the first sight. I watched her closely at Professor Tombak's lectures. During the first two days she had visible doubts about what was going on and she took no notes. On the third day her skepticism disappeared and she got busy with her pen and notebook. Later she performed the liver cleansing procedure in an impeccable manner. Having taken all prescribed doses of oil and lemon juice, she got rid of excess bile from her intestinal tract as early as midnight. At 2 a.m. the first three liver stones were "delivered" (without pain of course), at 3 a.m. her basin contained large amounts of green rice-like material and a few larger chunks of sediment, and at 7 a.m. 30-40 large liver stones were produced. She left Szczyrk glowing with joy, lighter by 8.8lb (4kg), free of pain in her knees or hands, and without the sensation of heaviness in her liver.

I saw her again exactly two weeks after the end of the retreat, just before I started writing this article. She seemed to be a completely different person. Her skin complexion was beautiful, her smile radiant, and her hands free of swelling. The overall change in the condition of her health was incredible: blood pressure 110/72, cholesterol level 203.3mg/dL, and weight reduced by another 6.6lb (3kg). She suffered no more from constipation or headaches and her hands were in perfect order.

It has to be admitted that she worked hard for these results. She carried out a seven-day fast on her return from the retreat.

"I am grateful" – she said – "for your program, which helped me set course towards good health. There is no comparison between the way I feel now and the way I felt three weeks ago. Another benefit I consider equally important is my newly gained awareness that return to good health requires strong will and self-discipline. No doctor can achieve it for us. We have to repair ourselves, what we have damaged over the years."

These were three stories of participants in our liver-cleansing program. There are many interesting facts I have not mentioned about last two retreats. Is it not fascinating, for example, that strict fasting made it possible for insulin-dependent diabetics (there were three of them) to do without insulin? During the fasting days, the sugar level in their blood fell to the normal value. There were more surprises of that sort. They would deserve some attention from medical schools.

This was the third time I had the opportunity to watch patients taking part in liver-cleansing retreats and to observe how the procedure benefits their physical and psychological health. I have no doubts that the method originated by Professor Mikhail Tombak is the best way to prevent many serious liver problems, including cirrhosis.

Excerpts from the article "Clean up the Key to your Health" by Nina Grelli

When I reported half a year ago my (and other people's) observations and reflections regarding therapeutic retreats with Professor Mikhail Tombak, I included a group picture of the participants taken at the end of the retreat. Everybody was visibly relaxed, smiling, and joyful. Such was not the case on the first day of the therapy. Dr. Barbara Buczynska, responsible for conventional medicine, did not hide her apprehension when she examined the participants. She almost begged some of them not to go through with the liver-cleansing procedure at the end of the retreat and to limit the therapy to dieting and enemas. It turned out that among the participants there were cancer and heart by-pass patients, diabetics, people suffering from high blood pressure and other chronic health conditions. Only a few healthy ones came for preventative reasons. Today I regret not having taken a picture on the first day. It would be interesting to compare these two pictures.

Over the next few months following the retreat, the participants informed me about further perceived changes in the condition of their health. They bragged about liver-cleansing routines done on their own and showed their satisfaction with obvious and permanent betterment of their health.

When we were leaving, one of the participants told me in secret that she could not share in the general enthusiasm of the group. She was afraid that the therapy did not meet the expectations of her daughter, who was the youngest participant. However, during "Encounters with Natural Medicine", which accompanied the fifteenth "Closer to Health, Closer to Nature" fair, I saw both of them smiling and happy. The mother informed me that her daughter (my favorite participant

242

in the retreat) has better appetite, sleeps better, does not suffer headaches anymore, and feels much healthier in general. The girl's appearance was totally different from the way she had looked several
months ago.

"There is nothing strange about it." – said Professor Mikhail
Tombak when I relayed to him on the phone my conversation with the
two women – "Sometimes the improvement happens immediately,
sometimes it takes a bit of time, but there is always a positive effect of
liver cleansing, which in turn results in a thorough cleanup of our entire body. Even with proper nutrition" – he stressed – "most of us do
not usually have the adequate level of necessary vitamins, enzymes,
micro-, and macroelements. We think, for example, that we take in
enough vitamin A because we drink carrot juice, eat red vegetables,
and even take betacaroten, but all of a sudden our eyesight becomes
worse. This means that something wrong is happening with our liver,
which is the main filter in our body. The filter is simply plugged."

"This can happen easily as a result of inflammations, infections,
stress, troubles, anger, diet rich in meat, smoked products, hot spices,
coffee, and alcohol, or the habit of eating large suppers. There may be
tens of causes that bring one result: provitamin A in our food passes
through our body as if in transit, without stopping. This means that our
body has no opportunity to synthesize vitamin A. There is a Chinese
saying, 'eyes are the liver's flower.' In our situation, the 'flower' starts
wilting – our eyesight becomes weaker, and not only the eyesight. Vitamin A deficiency also means poorer functioning of our heart and the
entire circulatory system, decreased supply of oxygen (nutrients) to
our brain, poor hormonal system function, etc. A similar thing happens
with vitamin E, commonly called the youth vitamin and related to vitamin A. This is exactly why liver problems can cause premature aging
and can be read directly from the sufferers' faces. "

"Liver cleansing is the base of our therapy, but the effects go
farther than the liver." – Professor Mikhail Tombak emphasizes –
"When we improve the functioning of our body's main laboratory,
we initialize the process of cleansing in our entire body, the process
of healing and rejuvenating. After the therapy, we soon notice an
improvement in the functioning of the entire digestive system, especially the pancreas, small and large intestine, better functioning of
our heart and the entire circulatory system, better functioning of our
brain, and an increased ability to deal with negative emotions, stress,

etc. This is why liver cleansing allows us to achieve good health results in amazingly short time.

To summarize, our liver is the key to our health. Its condition determines the state of our entire body and mind."

For more articles and other information visit **www.starthealthylife.com.**

APPENDIX C

Recipes for Health

Tibetan recipes for maintaining a youthful appearance

> To maintain clear whites of the eyes and a velvety shine, drink 1.8oz (50g) of parsnips juice every day.

> To prevent your eyes from shrinking as you age, massage your little fingers before sleep.

> As you age, you may become long-sighted and need glasses. To prevent this from happening, massage your index fingers, each 3 minutes a day.

> There is a good custom in the East called "Joy of the feet" – couples massage each other's feet. That is where we have over 70,000 nerve endings. Such massage removes fatigue, improves sleep, and extends longevity.

Preventing facial wrinkles

> **Recipe:** Blend 1 egg yolk, 1 tablespoon of glycerin, and 1 tablespoon of honey.
> **Usage:** Make a facial mask every morning and evening (10-15 minutes).

> **Recipe:** Grate a lemon with its peel and blend with 3.5oz (100g) of honey in a glass vessel.
> **Usage:** Make a facial mask once a day (10-15 minutes).

> **Recipe:** Blend 3.5oz (100g) of honey with 3.5oz (100g) of warmed-up vodka in a glass vessel.
> **Usage:** Warm up slightly and use as a facial mask once a day (15 minutes).

> **Recipe:** Cook a bunch of parsley in 0.5 quart (0.5 L) of water for 30 minutes, let it stand in room temperature for 30 minutes, strain, pour into a jar with a tight lid, and keep in a dark place for 2 days.
> **Usage:** Rub on your face every morning and evening; do not rinse off.

Removing facial wrinkles and spots

> **Recipe:** Chop up well 3.5oz (100g) of parsnips, put it in a pot, pour boiling water over it, and cook for 15 minutes. Let it stand in room temperature for 20 minutes, strain, blend with 1 tablespoon of lemon juice, and store in a dark place. **Usage:** Wash your face every morning and evening.

Healthy Cuisine Recipes

Homemade cheese low in casein and acids

Prepare 1 quart (1L) of skimmed milk, 7oz (200g) of kefir, 2.1oz (60g) of cream, and a flat teaspoon of baking soda. Boil the milk and, stirring constantly; pour kefir and cream in it. When it coagulates, add baking soda and strain water out.

Yeast-free bread

Mix four cups of flour with 0.5 quart (0.5L) of mineral water and work the dough until it does not stick to your fingers anymore. Form the dough into a loaf, heat up the oven and put the dough in it. Bake in 212-302F (100-150C) temperature. You can use a stick to check if the bread is ready. Keep the bread in the refrigerator – it will always feel soft and fresh.

Sweet bread

Mix 1.1lb (0.5kg) of flour with 1.8oz (50g) of oil, 1.8oz (50g) of honey, and 0.5 a cup of water make dough from it, and bake the same way as yeast-free bread. Keep refrigerated.

Healthy candy for children

Put some dried plums, figs, and apricots in warm water and soak them for 6-8 hours, take them out of the water, and stuff with walnuts (you can also dip them in honey and put bran on top of them).

Candy bars for children

Grind 0.9oz (25g) of roasted sunflower seeds, 0.9oz (25g) of raisins, 0.9oz (25g) of dried plums, 2 figs, and 0.9oz (25g) of walnuts. Mix the grinds and add 2 tablespoons of honey. Put into a form and keep in the refrigerator for 12 hours, then cut into bars. Store refrigerated.

A healthy dessert for adults and children

Grate about 5.3oz (150g) of apples, squeeze juice from 0.5 orange, add 10 walnuts and 2 teaspoons of honey, and mix everything well.

Universal recipes for seasoning soups, salads, meat, etc.

Blend 1 cup of kefir with juice from 3 garlic cloves - this makes a very tasty and healthy seasoning. Most people avoid garlic because of its odor. It can be removed by eating chopped-up parsley or a few slices of apple, lemon, or grapefruit.

Spring salads

1. **Radish and walnuts**
   Chop up or grate 15 radishes 3.5oz (100g), mix with 8 ground walnuts (1.4oz/40g), add 1 teaspoon of vegetable oil and put some chopped chive on top.

2. **French salad**
   Pour half a tablespoon of apple cider vinegar or wine vinegar over 3.5oz/100g of lettuce, add 1 tablespoon of vegetable oil and 1 teaspoon of chopped onion; mix everything well.

3. **Young beet salad**
   Grate five or six young beets, add 2 tablespoons of cream, and season with a pinch of ground cumin.

4. **Chive with peanuts**
   Chop up 1.8oz (50g) of chive and mix with 1.8oz (50g) of ground peanuts.

5. **Radish with nuts, parsley, and mint**
   Grate 15 radishes, add a chopped parsley, some mint and dill, 0.5 of cumin, and 6 tablespoons 1.8oz (50g) of ground nuts. Mix everything well. You can add some lettuce leaves as decoration.

6. Spinach salad
Chop up a handful of young spinach; add 1 tablespoon of chopped sorrel and 1 tablespoon of chopped chive; mix everything well. Add 3 tablespoons of ground peanuts and 1 tablespoon of bilberry.

7. Spinach and eggs
Whip up an egg yolk, gradually adding butter (1.5 tablespoon), then add 1 tablespoon of lemon juice. It should form a thick pulp when mixed. Add crushed garlic clove and 2 handfuls of chopped spinach. Mix again and put on a lettuce leaf.

8. Salad from beet leaves
Chop up young beet leaves (2 handfuls or about 2.1oz/60g). Prepare the sauce: Mix 1 egg yolk with 1 tablespoon of lemon juice, 0.5 teaspoon of mustard, 1 tablespoon of vegetable oil, and 1 teaspoon of chopped chive.

Summer and fall salads

1. Cucumbers and tomatoes
Mix chunks of cucumber with tomato slices; put 4 tablespoons of ground nuts on top.

2. Fresh cabbage salad
Mix 3.5oz (100g) of chopped cabbage with four tablespoons of grapefruit juice, 1 tablespoon of honey, and 0.5 teaspoon of cumin.

3. Peas and tomatoes
Mix 1.8oz (50g) of fresh peas with 4.2oz (120g) of crushed raw tomatoes and 2 tablespoons of sunflower oil. Put chopped parsley greens and chives on top.

4. Peas and carrots
Grate a carrot and mix it with 1.8oz (50g) of peas, 1 tablespoon of vegetable oil, 1 tablespoon of raspberry or currant juice, and chopped-up 0.5 of an onion.

5. Carrot with chive

Mix 3.5oz (100g) of grated carrots with 1.1oz (30g) of finely chopped chive; add 1 tablespoon of vegetable oil and put some finely chopped cucumber on top.

6. Blood-cleansing salad

Grate 1.8oz (50g) of beets and 1.8oz (50g) g of carrots; add 1.8oz (50g) of chopped cabbage, 1.5 tablespoon of olive oil, and 1.5 tablespoons of honey. Mix everything well and put a cupful of berries or red currant on top.

7. Cabbage with cumin

Chop up finely 3.5oz (100g) of cabbage; add 1 tablespoon of honey and 1 teaspoon of ground cumin

8. Tomatoes with carrot and nuts or biscuits

Crush 3.5oz (100g) of tomatoes and mix with 3.5oz (100g) of grated carrots, 1.1oz (30g) of chopped parsley, and 1.8oz (50g) of ground nuts or biscuits. Add 1.5 tablespoon of olive oil and mix again.

9. Salad from green beans

Remove the fibers from 2.1oz (60g) of young and tender bean pods and chop the pods finely. Add 1.8oz (50g) of lettuce chopped into larger pieces and 2 tablespoons of sunflower oil (you can also add 1 teaspoon of honey for better taste).

10. Pumpkin salad

Grate a carrot, 1.8oz (50g) of pumpkin, and 0.9oz (25g) of celery. Add 0.9oz (25g) of chopped chive or red onion and 1 ground nuts.

Winter salads

1. Beets and nuts

Grate a cooked large beet and 0.5 of a raw small beet. Add 1 crushed garlic clove and 1 tablespoons of vegetable oil. Mix everything well and put some ground nuts and a pinch of chopped chive on top.

2. Vitamin-rich salad
Grate 1.8oz (50g) of carrots, 2.6oz (75g) of cabbage, and 1.8oz (50g) of potatoes. Add 0.9oz (25g) of chopped parsley, 0.9oz (25g) of leek, 2 tablespoons of vegetable oil, 1 tablespoon of honey, and 1.8oz (50g) of ground nuts. Mix everything well.

3. Carrot and horseradish salad
Grate a large carrot and 1.8oz (50g) of celery roots. Add 1 tablespoon of grated horseradish, 0.35oz (10g) of ground nuts, and 1 tablespoon of vegetable oil. Mix everything well.

4. A holiday salad
Take a small red or white cabbage 2.6oz (75g) and chop it finely.
Add 0.5 of a grated average-sized carrot, 0.5 of a pickled cucumber, a 4-inch/10cm long finely chopped leek stem, 5 ground walnuts, 1 tablespoon of vegetable oil, and 3 tablespoons of oat cereal. Mix everything well.

Sauces and mayonnaises

Store-bought sauces and mayonnaises usually contain preservatives, coloring agents, and other substances foreign for our body and polluting our blood. This is why it is a good idea to prepare them on our own.

1. Lemon oil
Gradually add juice from 1 or 2 lemons as you stir 0.9oz (25g) of vegetable oil.

2. Nut mayonnaise (best prepared directly before the meal)
Mix 2 tablespoons of ground nuts with 1 teaspoon of vegetable oil to make a thick pulp. Then add 3-4 tablespoons of vegetable oil and whip it while gradually adding juice squeezed from 1 lemon.

3. Cream sauce
Mix juice from 0.5 lemon with 3 tablespoons of cream. Add a crushed garlic clove, 0.5 teaspoon of finely chopped chive or

grated onion, and 1 tablespoon of vegetable oil. Mix everything well.

4. Tomato sauce
Mix 6 parts of vegetable oil with 1 part of lemon juice. Blend it with tomato juice and add some grated celery for better taste.

5. "Rainbow" – a vitamin-rich mayonnaise
Whip 2 egg yolks while slowly adding 3 tablespoons of vegetable oil. Mix it with 1 tablespoon of grated celery or 1 teaspoon of grated onion and add some lemon juice. Whip well until it reaches normal mayonnaise thickness. You can color it green (with spinach juice), orange (with carrot juice), or pink (with red currant juice).

Desserts

1. Apple snow
Grate 2 or 3 apples and add 1 tablespoon of honey dissolved in 1 tablespoon of water. Mix it well. Separately, whip 2 egg whites while slowly adding some lemon juice. Mix everything together and whip again. Finally, you can decorate it with canned peaches, pears, frozen strawberries, fresh raspberries, or currants (use your imagination).

2. Apple web
Whip 2 egg yolks and 2 egg whites separately. Mix them and whip again. Dissolve 1 tablespoon of honey in 1 tablespoons of warm water. Grate 3 sweet apples and add 2 teaspoons of lemon juice to them. Mix everything together and whip again. Decorate with fresh fruits – berries, chunks of orange or grapefruit.

3. Honey cake
Mix 1.05oz (30 g) of lemon juice with 2.1oz (60g) of ground walnuts or peanuts. Let it stand for half an hour, and then add 2 tablespoons of honey and 2.1oz (60g) of ground rice. Mix everything and form into cakes. Put some ground roasted sunflower seeds on top.

Can We Live 150 Years?

Food products necessary for proper functioning of our brain:

Apricots	Apples	Cabbage	Carrots
Nuts	Cherries	Brussels sprouts	Celery
Grapefruits	Currants	Cauliflower	Cucumbers
Honey	Corn oil	Mint	Garlic
Raspberries	Olive oil	Horseradish	Liver
Parsley	Sunflower oil	Gooseberries	Oranges
Potatoes	Raisins	Grapes	Wheat sprouts
Peas	Raw egg yolk	Lettuce	Dried plums
Onion			

APPENDIX D

External Warning Signs of Internal Disorders

Dear readers, I would like you to pay attention to certain signs of diseases beginning in your body that can give you a warning before a medical diagnosis detects the disease. Watch for these signs no matter whether you feel ill or healthy. This will help you avoid unpleasant surprises that could damage your health.

Nonetheless, I want to stress that a physician should do the final diagnosis of a disease. Your own observation of the way your body behaves is only intended to help your physician in the task of making the diagnosis.

Since there are great variety of disorders and their warning signs, I am going to present the most common ones.

Disorders	External warning signs
Anemia	Pale face, brownish lower eyelid, pearl-colored sclera (the white of the eye), pearl-colored teeth, pale ears, sores in the corners of the mouth, burning sensation on the tongue, smooth and red tongue surface
High blood pressure	Red nose with lumps and visible tiny veins, eyebrows joined together, red cheeks
Low blood pressure	Pale face or its fragments, pale forehead, hanging eyelids

Frequent headaches	Joined eyebrows, wrinkles on one side of the forehead, a vertical wrinkle between eyebrows
Hemorrhoids	A deep dimple in the middle of the chin, yellow stains on the teeth
Liver inflammation	Yellow sclerotic coats of the eyes, yellow skin on the body or around the mouth, sunken cheeks, and tiny veins visible on the sides of the nose, brown skin around the eyes, white spots on the nails, expanded lower lip.
Gastritis	White residue on the middle section of the tongue, pale sides of the nose
Diabetes	Dry, smooth, bluish-red lower lip, some dead hair, premature graying
Predisposition to diabetes	Dry and chopped tongue, narrow upper lip
Pancreas overworked to an unhealthy degree	Wrinkled face, narrow upper lip
Prostate inflammation	Strongly expanded lower lip, pale-pink skin around the eyes

Unhealthy strain on the thyroid gland	Bulged nails, short eyebrows (missing the outer parts), frequent blinking residue on lower eyelids, swollen neck narrow nose. tops of the ears unnaturally folded
Weak functioning of female reproductive glands	Hair above the upper lip, rounded winkles on the forehead, thick bushy eyebrows
Sensitive stomach	Pointed nose
Stomach cramps	Hunched posture when walking
Other stomach disorders	Misshaped middle fingernails breaking fingernails
Circulatory disorders	White tip of the nose, joined eyebrows, early graying, pale face, pale lips, thick nails, flat occiput (back part of the head)
Lung disorders	Both shoulders shifted back, red cheeks, long neck frequent nose bleeds bulged fingernails
Painful or irregular menstrual cycles	Thin eyebrows
Vitamin A deficiency	Inability to produce tears while weeping, inability to see anything while entering a dark room

Vitamin B deficiency	Swollen tongue
Iron deficiency	Lower eyelids bluish and caved in, occasional white spots on the nails, red ears, frequent sores in the corners of the mouth
Calcium deficiency	Shiny skin on the ears
Magnesium deficiency	Twitching lower eyelids, surge of energy after 8 p.m., red skin around the nose
Deficiency in minerals	Breaking of the nails
Estrogen deficiency in women	Thin eyebrows
Overworked nervous system	Difficulties while climbing stairs (especially at a young age)
Metabolic disorders	Residue on lower eyelids, white spots on the nails
Predisposition to obesity	Rounded thick ears, very thick earlobes
To much tension on the body, fatigue	Small ears
Digestive disorders	Grooves along the nails, skin pimples, red ears
Frequent spine pain, spine disorders	Flat occiput, wide walking – swaying to the sides
Degenerated cervical vertebrae	Deep wrinkle by the right eyebrow

Lower sexual drive in men	Vertical wrinkles under the ears
The beginning of menopause in women	Many small deep wrinkles above the upper lip
Kidney disease	Large and thick upper lip, thick and wrinkled skin on the forehead, red lips, swollen lower eyelids, narrow and bulged nails with permanent white spots, bags under the eyes
Disorders of the gallbladder	Yellow skin around the mouth and eyes, yellow teeth, pains in the area of the right shoulder blade, yellowish eyes
Bladder disorders	Swollen, bluish-pink lower eyelids, unusually short body
Rheumatism	Foamy streaks on both sides of the tongue
Predisposition to rheumatism	Left shoulder higher than the right, pointy cave-ins on the nails
Inefficient heart function, other heart disorders	Swollen and waxy-looking lower eyelids, expanded veins on the neck, short neck, short nose, difficulties while climbing stairs
Predisposition to heart attacks	Wrinkled earlobes; The area between the lower lip and the chin gets numb when pressed

Sclerosis	Visible veins on the palms; The palms cannot be straightened flat.
Thrombosis (blood clots)	Visible broken blood vessels around the nose
Bad cholesterol balance	Round brown lumps (similar to warts) on the upper eyelid
Predisposition to epilepsy	Joined eyebrows
Predisposition to stomach ulceration	Narrow, split tip of the nose
Stomach ulcer	Pain in the left shoulder blade, white tip of the nose

APPENDIX E

Biological rhythms and your skin

The health of our skin is influenced by zodiac signs, but it also depends on the condition of our digestive organs such as the large intestine. This is why, regardless of what stars you were born under, cleanse your body and especially your large intestine and liver from time to time. In other words, learn about the stars but do your part of the job.

All physiological processes happening in our body are influenced by the Sun and the planets (cosmic rhythms). People born in different times of the year undergo specific changes on their skin depending on the zodiac sign they were born under.

Aries

The skin of an Aries is predisposed to inflammations and pus formation. Being impatient, people born under this sign damage the skin on their faces while trying to remove every new little pimple, often by squeezing it. They can benefit from moisturizing facial masks from tomatoes, strawberries, apples, carrots, etc. – any fruits or vegetables with high vitamin A and B content.

Taurus

Women born under this sign should pay particular attention to the skin on their neck – it is their weak side. The skin of a Taurus in general is prone to allergies and excessive sweating. Skin care should involve the use of moisturizing vitamin masks – from wild strawberries, cucumbers, bananas, and carrots with some olive oil. Hay, table salt, or sea salt are recommended to be added to the bathwater. After taking alternate hot and cold showers, they should rub an extract of sage, oak bark, or green tea on their skin. The skin on the neck needs particular attention. To keep it looking young, an alternate compress can be used once a week: 3 minutes hot and one minute cold, repeated 2-3 times. It is helpful to massage the front of the neck (for example while watching TV) top down using a regular tablespoon lubricated with some warm vegetable oil.

Gemini

People born under this sign tend to be of distrustful nature with little regard for a regular rhythm of life. They are so absorbed with their work that there is little time left for taking care of their health. Their skin is pretty dry and prone to scaling. They should pay particular attention to the skin on their arms and hands. Masks prepared from kiwi fruits, bananas, eggs, cottage cheese, or yeast are recommended. It is a good idea to add an herbal brew (one tablespoon of any herbs e.g. sage, nettle, etc. infused in 0.5 quart/L of water).

Cancer

Women born under this sign like to take care of their appearance on their own – they do not trust beauty salons. However, they could benefit a lot from physiotherapeutic procedures, especially massage. They have a very delicate skin that needs much care. It is best to use an herbal brew made from mint, chamomile, lime-tree blossom, or thyme. People born under the sign of Cancer have a predisposition for allergies and swelling. They can brew birch leaves or buds and make compresses to remedy this problem. To nurture and rejuvenate the skin, facial masks made from cabbage, cucumber, or rye bread can be used.

Leo

Female Leos always want to be beautiful and create a strong impression. Excessive taste for sweets often results in various pimples on their face. Blood vessels tend to expand and tiny veins show on the skin surface. They are highly sensitive to ultraviolet rays and should not expose their skin to direct sunlight too much – it is better to spend more time in the shade. Leos rarely suffer from allergies and their skin is healthy in most cases. Facial masks from potatoes, bananas, or watermelons are beneficial. To nurture the skin, creams containing almond and coconut milk are the best.

Virgo

The skin of people born under this sign reflects the condition of their intestines. Various rashes, pimples, and skin irritations are the results of digestive tract inflammations or constipation. All Virgos have a very sensitive stomach and must be careful with their diet. A diet rich in plant-based products helps keep a fresh and young appearance of the skin. Recommended masks are those made from apples, oat, and squash. Good remedies against constipation are juices from beets and apples, dried fruits soaked for 5-8 hours.

Libra

The skin of Libras is sensitive, prone to allergies, dry, and predisposed to early aging. Attention should be paid to the area around the eyes because it tends to be affected by dark rings and swelling, especially in times of nervous frustration. Moisturizing masks from wild strawberries, peaches, or cucumbers are recommended. It is helpful to drink a glass of cold mineral water before bedtime.

Scorpio

The skin of Scorpios is often afflicted with different pus rashes, mostly around the lips and on the nose. Moisturizing facial masks made from apples and cherries as well as conditioning facials based on cottage cheese and eggs are beneficial. It is a good idea to add brew from blackcurrant and mint to the bath water. The body of a Scorpio needs a high intake of vitamins B, C, and E.

Sagittarius

A Sagittarius often has an oily and porous skin with greenish discolorations. Cucumbers and grapes can be used to prepare facials. For bathing, brews from leaves of blueberry, raspberry, or parsley can be used. Because people born under this sign have a sensitive liver, they often suffer from furunculosis (recurring boils).

Capricorn

The main problems are: predisposition to allergies, dryness and scaling of the skin, and warts. The skin needs toning procedures. It is best to use boiled or mineral water for washing in case of skin problems. Recommended moisturizing masks are the ones made from cabbage, spinach leaves, or egg yolks. Capricorns should take particular care of their teeth and use their index finger with some toothpaste on it rather than a toothbrush for cleaning. This will provide a gum massage and prevent their delicate teeth from developing gum disease.

Aquarius

An Aquarius does not usually have skin problems, except that frequent stress and nervous strains can cause eczemas and itchy spots. Therefore, it is important to be able to control emotions and relax more frequently. Moisturizing facials from oranges, grapefruits, lemons, and watermelons are advised. The skin needs a high intake of vitamin D and B.

Pisces

People born under this zodiac sign have sensitive skin, prone to swelling and allergies. Masks made from carrots, wild strawberries, cucumbers, and grapes can moisturize the skin. A brew of sage or wormwood can be used as a skin cleanser. Body and face massages help maintain the skin in a good condition.

INDEX

Buckwheat, 109, 130
  preparing of, 106
Burns, 228-229, 231
Butter, 103
  remove additives from, 107, 123
Buttermilk, 103,

C

Cabbage juice, 86
Calcium, 20, 22, 23-24, 82,
  causes of calcium deficiency, 148,
    160
  child gender and, 171-172
  coffee and, 137
  forms of, 159,
  retaining, 164, 230
  sources of, 87, 130, 163
  unneeded, 80, 91, 93-94, 153
Cancer, 31, 35, 61, 71, 120, 235
  diet and, 36, 126
  fasting and, 60
  fried food and, 106
  heavy metals and, 208
  large intestine and, 183
  lead to, 20, 27, 39, 94,
  preventing, 83,127-130, 166-168,
    209
  structured water and, 80
Cardiovascular disorders
  treating, 223-226
Carrot juice, 85-86
Cataracts
  (See eyes cleansing)
Cholesterol, 23, 129, 153, 157
  lower, 67, 68, 89, 205
  pure butter and, 107, 123
Chronic diseases, 31, 111
  lemon therapy and, 161-163
Circulatory system cleansing, 202, 205,
  207, 209

Clover juice, 87-88
Coffee, 81-82
Colds, 69, 77,
  breathing and, 74
  causes of, 102
  colds prevention, 90, 96, 98, 99, 164
  frequent, 17, 21, 45, 76
  mucus and, 23
  nose cleansing and, 180-181
  synthetic vitamin C and, 170
  treating of, 216, 217
Colic, 87
Colon cancer
  lead to, 166
Complexion, 78, 84, 119, 120
  cleansing and, 208
Constipation, 34, 35, 172, 187
Causes of, 24, 27, 37, 80, 165
  get rid of, 80, 88, 92, 164, 177, 221
  prevention of, 165,
Copper, sources of, 163
Coughing treating, 215-218
Cramps, 92, 109
Cucumber juice, 87
Cysts, 61, 109

D

Dental, 148
Desserts, 109
Diabetes, 31, 103
  causes of, 20,
  remedy for, 86, 227
Diaphragm, 18, 33, 74, 182
Diet, 71, 78, 119, 121
  cancer and, 126, 127
  carbohydrates in, 105-106
  dairy products in, 24
  food groups in, 124
  gender of child and, 171-172
  healthy, 110-112, 125-126, 155-156

264

Healthy Life Press Inc.
145 Tyee Drive, PMB 355
Point Roberts, WA 98281-9602
USA

Email: orders@starthealthylife.com
Tel. (888) 575 3173
Fax: (604) 682 5817

"Can We Live 150 Years?" is available in English, Spanish, German, Polish, Korean and Romanian.
 Specify your language:_____

BOOK ORDER FORM

Please send ___ copies of the book *"Can We Live 150 Fears."*
at the price of:

    $19.95 US, for the total of...US $ _____

Please send ___ copies of the book *"Cure the Incurable"*
at the price of:

    $16.95 US, for the total of...US $ _____

Add Shipping and Handling:
(US $3.95 for one, add US $1.00 for each additional book)..US $ _____

    TOTAL...US $ _____

(Check applicable)
( ) Enclosed is my check or money order for US $ _____
( ) I would like to pay with my VISA

Shipping Address   Please Print Clearly

Your Name:	
Address:	
City, State/Province:	
Zip/Postal Code:	
Tel/Fax Number:	
Email address:	

Please charge my VISA Number:

Expiry Date:

		/	

The amount of .... US $ _____

Cardholder Name: _____

Signature: _____ Date: _____